Springer
Berlin
Heidelberg
New York
Barcelona
Budapest
Hong Kong
London
Milan
Paris
Santa Clara
Singapore
Tokyo

A.R. Damasio H. Damasio
Y. Christen (Eds.)

Neurobiology
of Decision-Making

With 62 Figures, Some in Color and 5 Tables

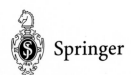 Springer

Damasio, A.R., M.D., Ph.D.
Department of Neurology
Division of Cognitive Neuroscience
The University of Iowa College of Medicine
Iowa City, IA 53342
USA

Damasio, H., M.D.
Department of Neurology
Division of Cognitive Neuroscience
The University of Iowa College of Medicine
Iowa City, IA 53342
USA

Christen, Y., Ph.D.
Fondation IPSEN
24, rue Erlanger
75781 Paris Cedex 16
France

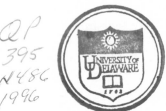

ISBN 3-540-60143-0 Springer-Verlag Berlin Heidelberg New York

Library of Congress Cataloging-in-Publication Data. Neurobiology of decision-making/A.R. Damasio, H. Damasio. Y. Christen (eds.). p. cm.—(Research and perspectives in neurosciences) Proceedings of a forum organized in Paris by the Fondation Ipsen. Includes bibliographical references and index. ISBN 3–540–60143–0 (hardcover: alk. paper) 1. Decision-making—Physiological aspects—Congresses. 2. Neuropsychology—Congresses. 3. Neurobiology—Congresses. I. Damasio, Antonio R. II. Damasio, Hanna. III. Christen, Yves. IV. Series. QP395.N486 1995 612.8′2—dc20 95–34650

© Springer-Verlag Berlin Heidelberg 1996
Printed in Germany

The use of general descriptive names, registered names, trademarks, etc, in this publication does not imply, even in the absence of a specific statement, that such names are exempt from the relevant protective laws and regulations and therefore free for general use.

Product Liability: The publishers cannot guarantee the accuracy of any information about dosage and application contained in this book. In every individual case the user must check such information by consulting the relevant literature.

Cover design: Springer-Verlag, Design & Production

Typesetting: Best-set Typesetter Ltd., Hong Kong

SPIN: 10482814   27/3132/SPS – 5 4 3 2 1 0 – Printed on acid-free paper

Introduction

Neuroscience has overlooked decision-making as much as it has neglected emotion, and even more so than it has resisted the study of consciousness. And yet the importance of decision-making is indisputable, especially in the context of the reasoning processes that culminate in the personal and social decisions that define rationality. Decision-making is, in fact, as defining a human trait as language. Interestingly, although no field has cohered around this topic to date, a variety of researchers in different areas of neuroscience – ranging from cellular physiology to neuropsychology and computational neuroscience – have been engaged in work that speaks directly to the issue. Thus, the time seemed ripe to bring together some of those researchers and discuss the state of the art in a broad forum that included the perspectives of normal cognitive psychology and physiology of mind. This book is a collection of the contributions presented at that forum (Colloque Médecine et Recherche: Neurobiology of Decision-Making, organized in Paris on October 24, 1994, by the Fondation Ipsen).

Iowa City, USA   *Antonio R. Damasio*
Iowa City, USA   *Hanna Damasio*
Paris, France   *Yves Christen*

Acknowledgments. The editors wish to thank Mrs Mary Lynn Gage for editorial assistance and Mrs Jacqueline Mervaillie for the organization of the meeting in Paris.

Contents

Feeling Reasons
P.S. Churchland

Epilogue: Models of Decision-Making
J. Altman

Contributors

Adolphs, R.
Department of Neurology, Division of Cognitive Neuroscience,
The University of Iowa College of Medicine, Iowa City, IA 52242, USA

Altman, J.
37D Lordship Park, London N16 5UN, Great Britain

Bechara, A.
Department of Neurology, Division of Cognitive Neuroscience,
The University of Iowa College of Medicine, Iowa City, IA 52242, USA

Berns, G.S.
Howard Hughes Medical Institute, Computational Neurobiology Laboratory,
Salk Institute for Biological Studies, P.O. Box 85800, San Diego, CA 92186-5800,
USA, and formerly Western Psychiatric Institute and Clinic, University of
Pittsburgh Medical Center, 3811 O'Hara Street, Pittsburgh, PA 15213, USA

Berthoz, A.
Laboratoire de Physiologie de la Perception et de l'Action,
Collège de France-CNRS, UMR 9950, Paris, France

Changeux, J.-P.
Institut Pasteur, 25, rue du Docteur Roux, 75015 Paris, France

Cherry, S.
Department of Molecular and Medical Pharmacology and Crump Institute
for Biological Imaging, UCLA School of Medicine, Los Angeles, CA 90024, USA

Christen, Y.
Fondation IPSEN, 24, rue Erlanger, 75781 Paris Cedex 16, France

Churchland, P.S.
Department of Philosophy, B-002, University of California, La Jolla, CA 92093,
USA

Damasio, A.R.
Department of Neurology, Division of Cognitive Neuroscience,
The University of Iowa College of Medicine, Iowa City, IA 52242, USA

Damasio, H.
Department of Neurology, Division of Cognitive Neuroscience,
The University of Iowa College of Medicine, Iowa City, IA 52242, USA

Dehaene, S.
Laboratoire des Neurosciences Cognitives, 54, Bld. Raspail, 75006 Paris, France

Fuster, J.M.
Department of Psychiatry and Brain Research Institute, School of Medicine,
University of California, 760 Westwood Plaza, Los Angeles, CA 90024, USA

Huang, S.-C.
Department of Energy, Laboratory of Structural Biology, UCLA, Los Angeles
CA 90024, USA, and Department of Molecular and Medical Pharmacology,
UCLA School of Medicine, Los Angeles, CA 90024, USA

Ingvar, D.H.
Department of Clinical Neurophysiology, University Hospital, 22185 Lund,
Sweden, and Department of Economic Psychology, Stockholm School
of Economics, 11383 Stockholm, Sweden

McGuire, M.
Department of Psychiatry and Brain Research Institute, UCLA,
School of Medicine, Los Angeles, CA 90024, USA,
and Nonhuman Primate Research Laboratory, Research Service,
Sepulveda Veteran Administration Medical Center, Sepulveda, CA 91343, USA

Melega, W.
Nonhuman Primate Research Laboratory, Research Service, Sepulveda Veteran
Administration Medical Center, Sepulveda CA 91343, USA, and Department
of Energy, Laboratory of Structural Biology, UCLA, Los Angeles, CA 90024, USA

Pandya, D.N.
Edith Nourse Rogers Memorial Veterans Administration Medical Center,
200 Springs Road, Bedford, MA 01730, USA, and Departments of Anatomy, and
Neurology, Boston University School of Medicine, Boston, MA 02118, USA

Phelps, M.
Nonhuman Primate Research Laboratory, Research Service, Sepulveda Veteran
Administration Medical Center, Sepulveda, CA 91343, USA, and Department
of Energy, Laboratory of Structural Biology, UCLA, Los Angeles, CA 90024, USA

Raleigh, M.
Department of Psychiatry and Brain Research Institute, UCLA School of Medicine, 760 Westwood Plaza, Los Angeles, CA 90024, USA, and Nonhuman Primate Research Laboratory, Research Service, Sepulveda Veteran Administration Medical Center, Sepulveda, CA 91343, USA

Sejnowski, T.J.
Howard Hughes Medical Institute, Computational Neurobiology Laboratory, Salk Institute for Biological Studies, P.O. Box 85800, San Diego, CA 92186-5800, USA

Sutherland, N.S.
Experimental Psychology, Biology Building, University of Sussex, Falmer, Brighton, BNI 9QG, Great Britain

Tranel, D.
Department of Neurology, Division of Cognitive Neuroscience, The University of Iowa College of Medicine, Iowa City, IA 52242, USA

Yeterian, E.H.
Edith Nourse Rogers Memorial Veterans Hospital, 200 Springs Road, Bedford, MA 01730, USA, and Department of Psychology, Colby College, Waterville, ME 04901, USA

Human Neuroanatomy Relevant to Decision-Making

H. Damasio

Reasoning and decision-making depend on large-scale neural systems that involve varied regions throughout the cerebral cortex and subcortical nuclei. The contributions in this volume, however, focus on a few of these regions, mostly in the frontal lobe. The purpose of this first chapter is to review the macroscopic anatomy of some of those structures.

Frontal Lobe Anatomy

Figures 1 and 2 depict a normal human brain seen from several perspectives. It is the brain of a living person shown in a three-dimensional reconstruction (3-D) from high-resolution magnetic resonance (MR) data, using the Brainvox[R] technique (Damasio and Frank 1992). It is apparent from these figures that the frontal lobe is not just the largest sector of the telencephalon but also the one with the clearest borders. Its limits are formed by clearly identifiable sulci. Posteriorly, the frontal lobe is separated from the parietal by the central sulcus, which has a supero-inferior and postero-anterior course. Inferiorly, the frontal lobe is separated from the temporal lobe by the sylvian fissure, a sulcus that runs antero-posteriorly in a slightly ascending direction. On the mesial surface the inferior limit is constituted by the callosomarginal sulcus, assuming we include the anterior sector of the cingulate gyrus in the frontal lobe instead of assigning it to a fifth lobe, the limbic.

Inspection of the lateral surface of the frontal lobe reveals the presence of several sulci and gyri. The precentral sulcus runs parallel and anterior to the precentral sulcus, with which it delimits the precentral gyrus. The inferior and superior frontal sulci have an antero-posterior course from the polar (most anterior) region of the frontal lobe towards the precentral sulcus. These two sulci are roughly parallel to each other and subdivide the lateral surface of the frontal lobe into inferior, middle and superior frontal gyri. The inferior frontal gyrus is traditionally known as the frontal operculum and is subdivided into three segments by the anterior rami of the sylvian fissure. The ascending ramus (the most posterior one) creates the anterior limit of the pars opercularis. The pars opercularis is the

Department of Neurology, University of Iowa College of Medicine, Iowa City, IA 52242, USA

A.R. Damasio et al. (Eds.)
Neurobiology of Decision-Making
© Springer-Verlag Berlin Heidelberg 1996

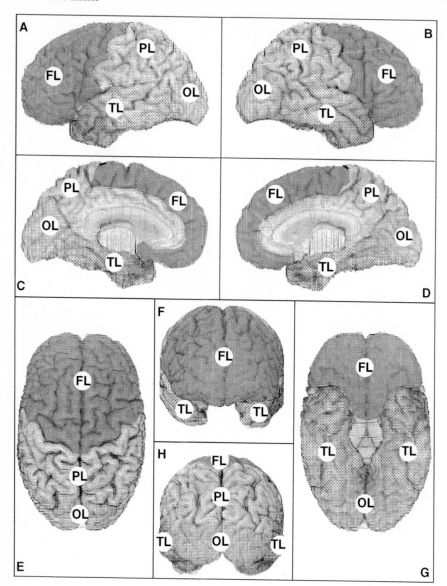

Fig. 1. Normal human living brain, reconstructed from 120 T₁ weighted consecutive coronal magnetic resonance slices (1.5 mm thick) using Brainvox, and seen from both the lateral (**A** and **B**) and mesial (**C** and **D**) views for both hemispheres, and from the superior (**E**), anterior (**F**), inferior (**G**) and posterior views (**H**). The frontal lobe (FL) is colored in red, the parietal lobe (PL) in green, the temporal lobe (TL) in blue and the occipital lobe (OL) in magenta. The cingulate gyrus is colored in yellow. It usually is divided between the frontal and parietal lobes when it is not considered part of a fifth lobe, the limbic lobe

posterior segment of the inferior frontal gyrus sitting between the ascending ramus and the inferior segment of the precentral sulcus. The horizontal ramus creates the antero-inferior border of the pars triangularis (the segment of the inferior frontal gyrus sitting between the two anterior rami of the sylvian fissure). The horizontal ramus also represents the superior border of the pars opercularis, which corresponds to the inferior and anterior segment of the inferior frontal gyrus, which blends into the orbital surface of the frontal lobe. The fronto-marginal sulcus runs horizontally across the polar region.

On the mesial aspect, the most notable sulcus is the cingulate sulcus, which runs parallel to the corpus callosum and separates the mesial sector of the superior frontal gyrus from the cingulate gyrus. At the juncture of the posterior third with the anterior two-thirds of the cingulate gyrus, the cingulate sulcus curves upward, forming the ascending branch of the cingulate sulcus. This sulcus is a useful landmark because it helps identify the mesial termination of the central sulcus, which usually lies just anterior to it.

On the inferior (orbital) surface of the frontal lobe we can see a prominent antero-posterior sulcus, roughly parallel to the interhemispheric fissure, the olfactory sulcus. It constitutes the lateral border of the gyrus rectus. Several other sulci can be seen lateral to this gyrus. They form an H-shaped image and are normally referred to as the orbital sulci. (For other comments on intrasubject and intersubject variability of the frontal lobe sulci and gyri, see H. Damasio 1995).

Traditionally, we consider three main sectors in the frontal lobe: the dorsolateral, the mesial and the orbital sectors (Fig. 3). There are, however, other ways of dividing this vast territory of the telencephalon. We can describe a motor sector (mostly the precentral gyrus), a premotor sector (the most anterior segment of the inferior half of the precentral gyrus, the posterior third of the superior and middle frontal gyri and the pars opercularis of the inferior frontal gyrus), and a prefrontal sector that encompasses all the remaining aspects of the frontal lobe. The pars triangularis can be considered as part of the premotor or the prefrontal sector (Fig. 3).

We now turn to cytoarchitectonic divisions (see Fig. 4a). The motor sector is occupied by Brodmann's field 4, on both the lateral and mesial surfaces. The premotor sector is constituted by Brodmann's fields 44 and 6. Field 6 continues into the mesial surface of the hemisphere, where it is usually designated as the supplementary motor area. Anterior to field 6, both on the lateral and mesial surfaces, is a band of yet another cytoarchitectonic area, field 8, which is also usually included in the premotor region.

The prefrontal region is made up of fields 45, 46, 9 and 10 on the lateral surface. These latter two fields (9 and 10) also extend into the mesial surface, where they are bordered by field 32. The sector of the anterior cingulate that may be considered to be in the frontal lobe is occupied by field 24. In the orbital sector we find fields 12, 11, 13, 25 and 47.

The vascular supply of the frontal lobe belongs to two distinct arterial territories, the anterior and middle cerebral arteries. The mesial surface of the frontal lobe is under the supply of the anterior branches of the anterior cerebral artery,

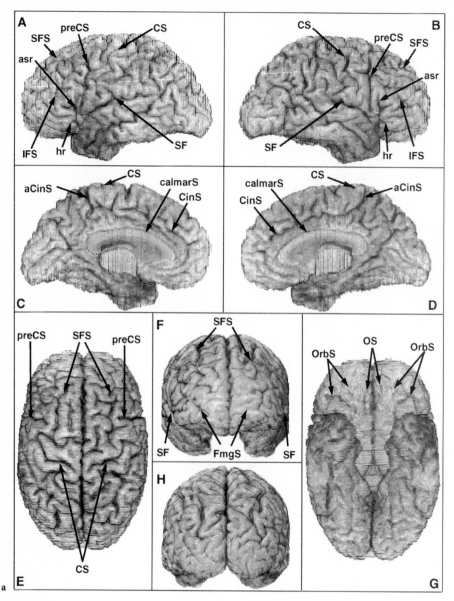

Fig. 2. Same brain as in Figure 1, seen from same views (**A-H**), with the major sulci and gyri of the frontal lobe marked in all views. **a** CS, central sulcus; preCS, precentral sulcus; SFS, superior frontal sulcus; IFS, inferior frontal sulcus; FmgS, frontomarginal sulcus; calmarS, callosomarginal sulcus; CinS, cingulate sulcus; aCinS, ascending branch of cingulate sulcus; OS, olfactory sulcus; OrbS, orbital sulci; SF, sylvian fissure; asr, ascending ramus of sylvian fissure; hr, horizontal ramus of sylvian fissure; **b** preCg, precentral gyrus; SFG, superior frontal gyrus; MFG, middle frontal gyrus; IFG, inferior frontal gyrus; paOp, pars opercularis; paTri, pars triangularis; paOrb, pars orbitalis (paOp + paTri + parOrb, frontal operculum or inferior frontal gyrus); PCL, paracentral lobule; SMA, supplementary motor area; FPole, frontal pole; Cing, cingulate gyrus; GR, gyrus rectus; OrbG, orbital gyri

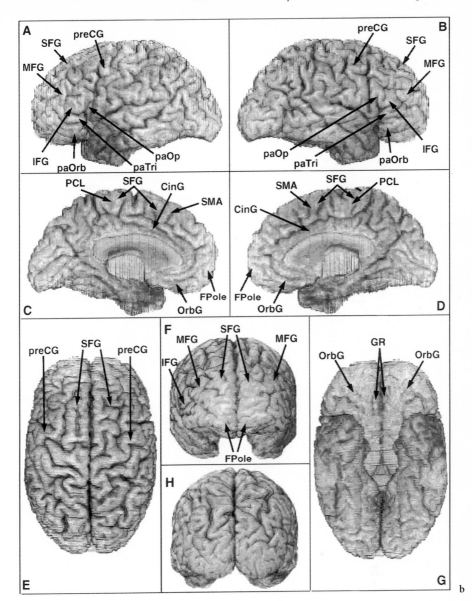

Fig. 2b

more specifically the frontopolar, anterior inferior, middle inferior and posterior inferior arteries, and the paracentral artery in the more posterior sector. The anterior pericallosal artery supplies blood to the corpus callosum and the inferior sector of the cingulate gyrus. The lateral surface of the frontal lobe is supplied by the anterior branches of the middle cerebral artery, the prefrontal, precentral and central arteries. The orbital surface is supplied by both the anterior and middle

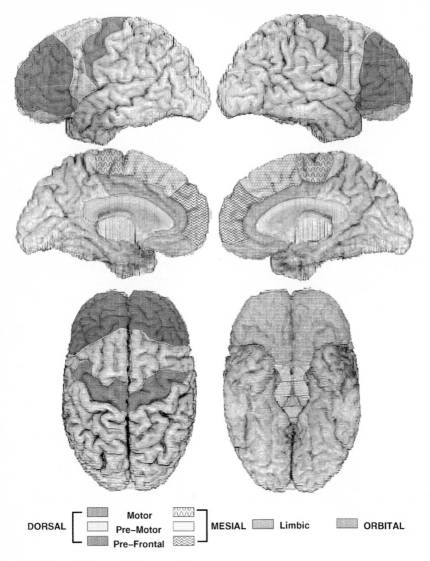

Fig. 3. Same brain seen in Figure 1 with grids identifying the different sectors of the frontal lobe

cerebral arteries through their orbitofrontal branches. The border zone between the two main vascular territories runs roughly along the lateral edge of the superior frontal gyrus (Fig. 4b).

Lesions in the Frontal Lobe

The most frequently encountered lesions affecting the frontal lobes fall into three main categories: vascular lesions, such as infarcts or hemorrhages; surgical

prefrontal regions and certain complex processes. For example, the caudal prefrontal region has been found to be involved in attentional mechanisms (e.g., Welch and Stuteville 1958; Heilman et al. 1970), whereas the ventrolateral prefrontal cortex appears to have a role in the regulation of response inhibition (e.g., Iversen and Mishkin 1970; Stamm 1973). As another example, while the dorsolateral prefrontal region is implicated in mnemonic processes (e.g., Passingham 1985; Funahashi et al. 1989), the ventromedial portion has been viewed as crucial to decision-making (Damasio et al. 1991). The existence of such structure-function relationships raises an important question: Are the discrete functions ascribed to prefrontal regions subserved intrinsically by these cortices, or do they depend upon interactions with other prefrontal areas? A more general issue concerns the extent to which the processes that are known to have a key focus within the prefrontal cortex also depend upon relationships with post-Rolandic and subcortical regions.

There is a significant amount of information available from neurobehavioral and neuroimaging studies in humans describing the localization of functions in the prefrontal cortex (e.g., Petersen et al. 1988, 1989; Petrides 1991; Damasio and Anderson 1993; Petrides et al. 1993a,b). Likewise, many neurophysiological and behavioral investigations in monkeys have established a number of similar structure-function relationships (e.g., Rosenkilde 1979; Fuster 1984; Bachevalier and Mishkin 1986; Wilson et al. 1993). However, although nonhuman primates have long served as important models for understanding the organization of the human brain, it is often difficult to interrelate the findings obtained from humans with those from nonhuman primates. One major factor in this regard is the lack of correspondence between architectonic schemas, making it difficult to specify which areas in the human and monkey prefrontal cortex are comparable. If these discrepancies were resolved, then clearer functional comparisons could be made with reference to specific architectonic regions. Moreover, in the light of recent proposals of functional cortical organization that emphasize the existence of dis-tributed neural networks (e.g., Goldman-Rakic 1987), the extensive connectional data that are available only for nonhuman primates could be extrapolated to the human brain. Therefore, in addressing a complex process such as decision-making from a neural point of view, it may be helpful to consider functional aspects in the context of the morphological features of the prefrontal cortex, in particular, architectonics and connections.

Architectonic Organization of the Prefrontal Cortex in Human and Monkey

Many investigators since the turn of the century have been attracted to the study of the cell and fiber organization of the human brain. The most commonly used map resulting from such inquiry is that of Brodmann (1909; Fig. 1). With specific regard to the prefrontal cotex, Figure 2 highlights the architectonic areas as delineated in the maps of Brodmann (1909), Economo and Koskinas (1925), and Sarkissov et al.

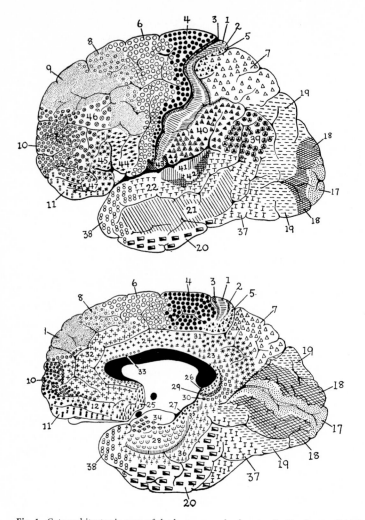

Fig. 1. Cytoarchitectonic map of the human cerebral cortex by Brodmann (1909)

(1955). These architectonic schemas reflect differences in the number and the extent of cortical areas. Despite the evident discrepancies in the delineations of certain prefrontal areas, there appears to be an overall commonality among the maps.

Similar architectonic maps have been generated for the prefrontal cortex of the monkey. The most widely used are those of Brodmann (1905; Fig. 3A,B); Vogt and Vogt (1919; Fig. 3C), Walker (1940; Fig. 3E), and Bonin and Bailey (1947; Fig. 3D). More recently, the prefrontal cortex has been parcellated by Matelli et al. (1985), Barbas and Pandya (1989), Preuss and Goldman-Rakic (1991), and Watanabe-Sawaguchi et al. (1991). Just as for the human maps, there are striking similarities as well as differences in areal demarcations.

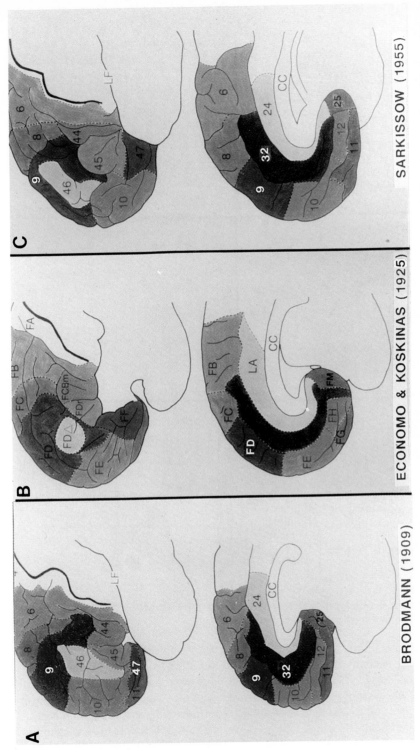

Fig. 2. Architectonic maps of the human frontal lobe showing equivalent architectonic areas, with specific colors used to facilitate the comparison of the boundaries of similar areas

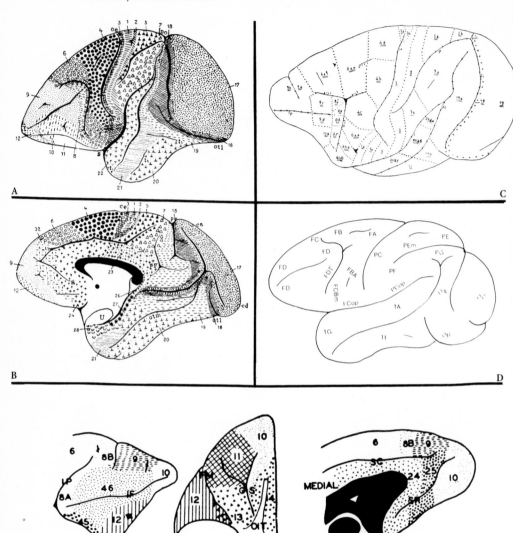

Fig. 3. Architectonic maps of the monkey cerebral cortex. **A** and **B** Brodmann (1905). **C** Vogt and Vogt (1919). **D** Bonin and Bailey (1947). **E** Walker (1940)

From a comparison of these architectonic maps of human and monkey prefrontal cortex, it becomes evident that there are numerous discrepancies both in the delineation of areas as well as in nomenclature. Therefore, it is often difficult to compare and to correlate clinical and experimental observations from humans with experimental data in monkeys. To obviate this problem, we have re-examined the architectonic organization of the prefrontal cortex in human and in macaque monkey (Petrides and Pandya 1995). The main aim of this work was to re-analyze the architectonic delineations in the brains of both species, and to look for specific relations and patterns among the areas. A second purpose was to refine the nomenclature so that areas that are indeed architectonically similar in both species have the same designation. Among the prefrontal cortices of both human and monkey, areas 24, 25, 32, and 10 as described by previous investigators are consistent in terms of location as well as nomenclature. In contrast, areas 44, 45, 8, 9, 46, 47, 12, 13, 11, and 14 differ significantly in terms of their designations and locations. In the following section, we will present an overview of our recent analysis with the aim of reconciling existing differences in the architectonic maps of these two species (Figs. 4 and 5). We will describe only the most salient features of prefrontal architectonic areas. A full description is presented by Petrides and Pandya (1995).

Architectonic Re-examination of the Prefrontal Cortex of Human and Monkey

Area 44

This area in the human brain is located in the pars opercularis, immediately rostral to area 6 (Fig. 4A). Architectonically, it is dysgranular in appearance; that is, it has a poorly developed layer IV and large pyramidal neurons in the deep portion of layer III. In the monkey brain, area 44 has not been delineated previously. However, our analysis has revealed the existence of an area with architectonic characteristics similar to those of area 44 in human, located within the caudal bank of the inferior limb of the arcuate sulcus (Fig. 5F). Thus, in both species, area 44 lies rostral to ventral area 6 and caudal to area 45.

In humans, area 44 is considered to be the major constituent of Broca's area, and is involved in various aspects of speech production. In monkeys, unlike area 6 neurons, which are strongly motor-related, neurons in area 44 are linked to goal-directed movements involving the hand or the mouth (Rizzolatti et al. 1988). Electrical stimulation of the cortex of the caudal bank of the arcuate sulcus results in simultaneous activation of different groups of laryngeal musculature, as opposed to stimulation of area 6, which results in the contraction of individual muscles of the larynx (Hast et al. 1974). Therefore, on architectonic as well as functional grounds, area 44 in both species may be involved in communication such as nonverbal vocalization and language.

Area 8

In both human and monkey, area 8 lies on the dorsolateral surface of the prefrontal cortex, rostral to dorsal area 6 and caudal to area 9, and extends medially into the superior frontal gyrus (Fig. 4A). In monkey, this area has been divided into two

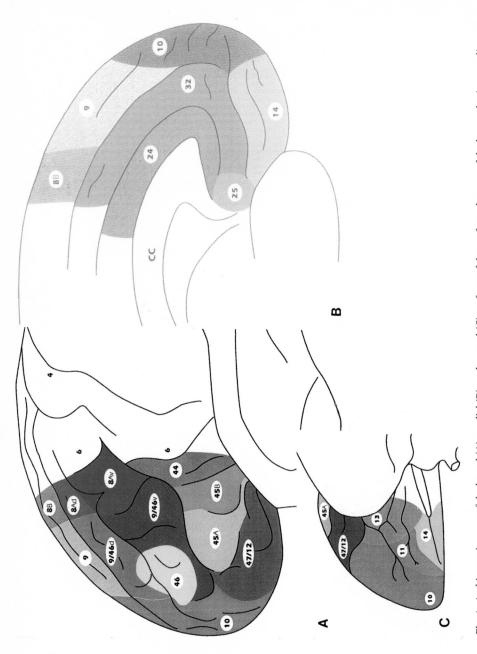

Fig. 4. Architectonic maps of the lateral (A), medial (B), and ventral (C) surfaces of the prefrontal cortex of the human brain according to Petrides and Pandya (1995)

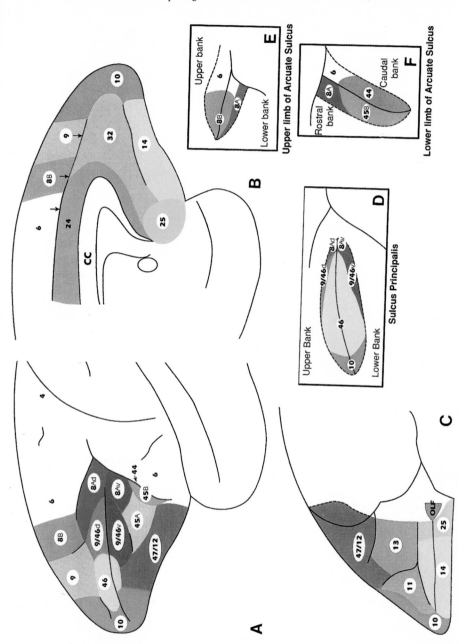

Fig. 5. Architectonic map of the lateral (**A**), medial (**B**), and ventral (**C**) surfaces of the macaque monkey brain according to Petrides and Pandya (1995). **D**, **E**, and **F** show the cortices in the depths of the principal sulcus, the upper limb of the arcuate sulcus, and the lower limb of the arcuate sulcus, respectively

parts, 8A in the arcuate concavity, and 8B extending dorsally from the arcuate region toward midline (Walker 1940; Fig. 3E). In the human prefrontal cortex, we have noted that in the ventral part of area 8 there is a well-developed layer IV and large pyramidal cells in layer III, whereas the dorsal and medial portion of area 8 has a less developed layer IV, with relatively few large pyramidal neurons in the lower part of layer III. Since similar features also distinguish the dorsal and ventral portions of area 8 in the monkey, we have designated the lower part of area 8 in human as 8A and the upper part as 8B. Area 8A in both species has been subdivided further into areas 8Ad (dorsal part) and 8Av (ventral part) because of subtle differences in architecture (Figs. 4A and 5A).

Area 45

This area in human is located in the pars triangularis and is characterized by a very well-developed layer IV and large pyramidal neurons in the lower part of layer III. In monkey, we have identified area 45 in the rostral bank of the lower limb of the arcuate sulcus, consistent with the observation by Walker (1940). However, we have noted that this area seems to extend farther rostrally into the ventrolateral frontal convexity, and that it has architectonic features that resemble those of area 45 in human. Moreover, as in the human brain, we have divided area 45 in monkey into two sectors, 45A rostrally and 45B caudally, on the basis of slight differences in architectonic characteristics (Figs. 4A and 5A).

Areas 9 and 46

The mid-dorsolateral sector of the prefrontal cortex contains two classically defined architectonic areas, 9 and 46, in both human and monkey (Figs. 2 and 3). However, whereas area 9 in human has been shown to surround area 46 (with the exception of the rostral portion of area 46), in monkey it is located dorsal to area 46. Several investigators, however, have suggested that there are architectonic subdivisions within both of these areas in monkey (Barbas and Pandya 1989; Preuss and Goldman-Rakic 1991). We have carefully re-examined the subregions of these areas specifically with the purpose of delineating possible commonalities in terms of morphological features. Accordingly, area 9, both in human and monkey, occupies the dorsalmost mid-portion of the lateral prefrontal cortex and extends medially up to the paracingulate (in human) and the cingulate (in monkey) sulcus (Fig. 4A,B, and Fig. 5A,B). Unlike the surrounding regions, the dorsal part of area 9 is dysgranular; that is, it has a poorly developed layer IV. Area 46 in human lies rostral to area 9 in and around the rostral portion of the middle frontal sulcus. This cortex is characterized by a well-developed layer IV as well as predominantly medium-sized pyramids in layers III and V. A similar region (area 46) in monkey is found in and around the rostral one-half of the principal sulcus, and extends caudally within both banks of that sulcus to area 8 (Fig. 5D). In human, the region that lies between areas 10 and 8, and essentially surrounds area 46, is characterized by a well-developed layer IV and a well-developed layer III that contains a significant number of large pyramidal neurons. This region classically is considered a part of area 9 (Fig. 4A). In monkey, the region between areas 46 and 8 surrounding the caudal part of the principal sulcus has architectonic features that are similar to part of the region just described in the human brain. This region traditionally has been considered a part of area 46. We have attempted to reconcile this discrepancy in nomenclature for these architectonically and topographically similar cortices by designating this region as area 9/46 in both human and monkey. Furthermore, we have divided this region into a dorsal sector, 9/46d, and a ventral sector, 9/46v.

Areas 47 and 12

In the human brain, Brodmann (1909) designated as area 47 a region ventral to area 45 and caudal to area 10 (Fig. 1). This area extends onto the orbital surface of the brain. A topographically similar region in the monkey brain was designated as area 12 by Walker (1940; Fig. 3E). Since these regions in both human and monkey have a basically similar architectonic pattern, we have labeled this region as 47/12 in both species to reconcile the previous inconsistency (Figs. 4 and 5).

Area 13

In monkey, the caudal part of the orbital frontal cortex located between the lateral and medial orbital sulci has been designated as area 13 by Walker (1940; Fig. 3E). In human, this cortical region has been subsumed as part of the orbital portion of area 47 (Fig. 1) rather than being designated as area 13. Our examination of this region in both species reveals common architectonic features, that is, a faint layer IV, and supra- and infragranular layers of approximately the same thickness. On the basis of the similarity in topography as well as morphology, we have designated this region in the human frontal lobe as area 13 (Fig. 4C).

Area 11

In monkey, area 11 is located rostral to area 13 and caudal to area 10 on the orbital surface of the frontal lobe (Walker 1940; Fig. 3E). In human, in contrast, the cortical region designated as area 11 has been shown to occupy the gyrus rectus on the ventromedial surface of the hemisphere (Fig. 1). As described below, we consider this portion of the frontal lobe in the human brain to be part of area 14. We have identified a region on the orbital surface of the human brain between areas 10 and 13 as area 11, because it has architectonic features similar to those of area 11 in monkey (Fig. 5C).

Area 14

In monkey, area 14 occupies the gyrus rectus and is bordered anteriorly by area 10 and posteriorly by area 25 (Fig. 3E). In human, as mentioned above, the cortex around the gyrus rectus has been considered as areas 11 and 12 (Fig. 1). Since the architectonic features of this topographic region in monkey and human are similar, we have designated this area as 14 in both species (Figs. 4B,C and 5B,C).

In the discussion above, we have focused on the areas of the frontal lobe about which there have been notable discrepancies when making comparisons between the human and monkey brain. There are other frontal cortical regions, however, namely areas 24, 25, 32, and 10, whose delineation has been more consistent in both species.

The existence of different architectonic areas within the prefrontal cortex of human and monkey raises the question of whether there is an underlying principle by which these cortical regions may be systematically interrelated. In the following section, we will discuss the organization of prefrontal areas with regard to laminar differentiation.

Architectonic Trends in the Prefrontal Cortex of Human and Monkey

Although the cortical maps described above may allow for comparisons between species, a consideration of discrete areas within an overall organizational framework may help to further our understanding of the contributions of the prefrontal cortex to higher-order processes. One approach to the architecture of the cerebral cortex in general has been to consider the diverse regions as belonging to one of two general groupings, or trends. These trends are considered to have distinctive sites of origin (according to the concept of a dual origin of the cerebral cortex) and to be characterized by sequential architectonic differentiation (Dart 1934; Abbie 1940; Sanides 1969; Pandya and Yeterian 1985). According to this conceptualization, one trend arises from the paleocortical (olfactory) moiety, whereas the other originates in the archicortical (hippocampal) moiety (Fig. 6A). From each of these moieties, a cortical architectonic trend can be traced, passing through periallocortex and proisocortex prior to culminating in true six-layered isocortex

Fig. 6. **A** Diagram of the basal surface of the cerebral cortex in the rhesus monkey showing the location of the two primordial moieties, olfactory cortex (paleocortical) and hippocampus (archicortical). **B** Flow diagram depicting cortical architectonic sequences emanating from the two primordial moieties. **C** Diagrammatic representation of the further progression of the two cortical evolutionary trends shown in Figure 4, culminating in pre- and post-Rolandic sensory and motor cortical areas (Pandya and Yeterian 1985). Abbreviations for this and other figures: A_I, primary auditory area; A_{II}, second auditory area; AS, arcuate sulcus; CC, corpus callosum; CF, calcarine fissure; CING S, cingulate sulcus; CS, central sulcus; G, gustatory area; HIPPO, hippocampus; IOS, inferior occipital sulcus; IPS, intraparietal sulcus; LF, lateral fissure; LS, lunate sulcus; M_I, motor cortex; M_{II}, supplementary motor area; OLF, olfactory cortex; OS, orbital sulcus; OTS, occipitotemporal sulcus; PALL, periallocortex; POMS, parieto-occipito-medial sulcus; Pro or pro-iso, proisocortex; Pro st, prostriate region; PS, principal sulcus; Rh F, rhinal fissure; S_I, primary somatosensory area; S_{II}, second somatosensory area; SSA, supplementary sensory area; STS, superior temporal sulcus; V_I, primary visual area; V_{II} (MT), second visual area; VS, vestibular area

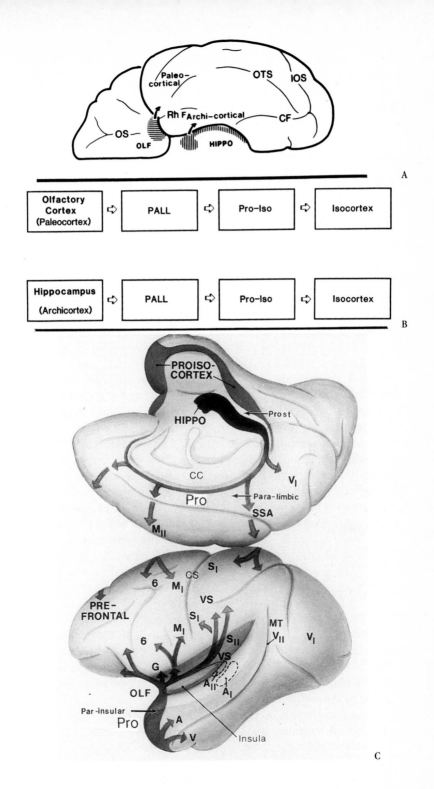

(Fig. 6B). The isocortical areas that stem from the paleo- and archicortical moieties show progressive laminar differentiation that can be followed from the proisocortex toward the primary sensory and motor regions as successive stages of elaboration of cortical laminae. This laminar differentiation occurs in each cortical layer; however, the overall pattern seems to show progressive development of supragranular layers as one moves from the proisocortex toward the primary regions. Thus, the temporal polar and insular proiocortices are viewed as being derived from the paleocortical moiety (Fig. 6C). Further progression from the proisocortices would lead to the development of auditory-related areas of the superior temporal region, the areas relating to the central visual field in the occipital and inferotemporal cortices, the somatosensory and motor areas subserving the head, face, and neck in the ventral part of the post- and precentral gyri, and the gustatory and vestibular areas. From this paleocortical trend also would evolve the various regions of the ventral prefrontal cortex. The proisocortices of the archicortical trend, which are located in the ventral temporal and cingulate regions, give rise to the ventromedial temporal and occipital areas subserving peripheral vision, and to somatosensory and motor areas relating to the trunk and limbs. From this medial proisocortical area also would evolve the medial and dorsolateral prefrontal regions.

This conceptualization provides a common framework for organizing prefrontal cortical areas in both monkey (Figs. 7 and 8) and human (Figs. 9 and 10) in a sequential manner. In describing the architectonic trends, we have used the new designations for human cortical areas as described above. However, for the monkey we have employed a recent modification of Walker's (1940) architectonic parcellation proposed by Barbas and Pandya (1989). Thus, in both the macaque and the human brain the paleocortical trend is viewed as having its origin in the proisocortex of the caudal orbital frontal region, which has an emphasis on infragranular layers but has no fourth layer. From the proisocortex, the next stage of differentiation is represented by areas 14, 11, 13, and orbital area 12, which have a predominance of infragranular layers but also have an incipient layer IV (Figs. 7A, 8A, and 9A). Progressing further within this trend, the next level of differentiation is composed of area 10, lateral area 12 (or 47/12), and the ventral portion of area 46 (Figs. 8A and 9B). These regions are characterized by an approximately equal emphasis on infra- and supragranular layers, and further development of layer IV. The paleocortical trend culminates in areas 9/46v (or caudal area 46), 8Av (or ventral area 8), 45, and 44, all of which have a predominance of supragranular layers, prominent pyramidal neurons in layer III, and a highly developed layer IV (Figs. 7, 8A, and 9C). Area 44, although it has a well-developed layer III, has a less elaborate layer IV, probably because it is related to the adjoining motor cortices as well as to the prefrontal region.

The archicortical trend is considered to have its origin in the allo- and periallocortices around the corpus callosum, which leads to the development of the proisocortices surrounding the rostrum of the corpus callosum, consisting of areas 25, 32, and 24 (Figs. 7B, 8B, and 10A). These areas have a predominance of infragranular layers, and virtually no layer IV. The next stage of differentiation is

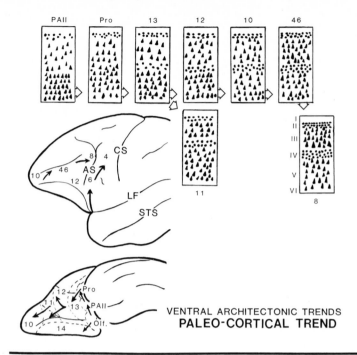

VENTRAL ARCHITECTONIC TRENDS
PALEO-CORTICAL TREND

A

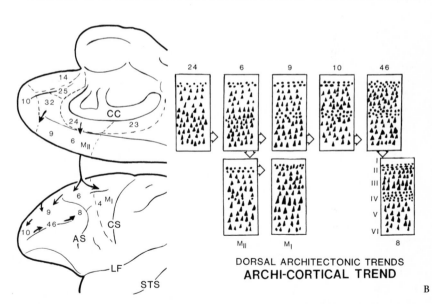

DORSAL ARCHITECTONIC TRENDS
ARCHI-CORTICAL TREND

B

Fig. 7. Diagrammatic representations of the progressive laminar organization of the areas of the prefrontal cortex in the rhesus monkey. **A** Paleocortical trend; **B** Archicortical trend

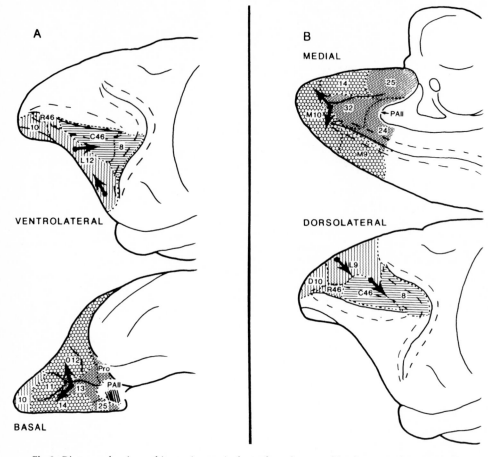

Fig. 8. Diagrams showing architectonic areas in the prefrontal cortex of the rhesus monkey arranged in stages within the orbital and ventral (**A**) as well as the medial and dorsolateral (**B**) regions, i.e., within the paleocortical and archicortical trends, respectively. Within each trend the axis of differentiation proceeds in a direction from the least differentiated periallocortex (PAll) to area 8, which represents the most highly elaborated cortex (Barbas and Pandya 1989)

represented by the medial division of areas 14, 10, 9, and 8B (Figs. 7B, 8B, and 10B). Each of these cortices can be described as dysgranular, containing an incipient fourth layer. The next areas in sequence consist of dorsolateral areas 9 and 10 and dorsal area 46, which have a well-developed fourth layer and an equivalence of infra- and supragranular layers (Figs. 7B, 8B, and 10C). Finally in this trend are areas 9/46d (or caudal area 46) and 8Ad (or dorsal area 8), which contain a highly developed layer IV and a predominance of supragranular layers (Figs. 7B, 8B, and 10D). Within specific stages of architectonic differentiation, each area has a unique morphological pattern. However, the overall features of areas within each stage are similar.

This conceptualization of dual architectonic trends within the cerebral cortex, in particular the prefrontal region, raises the issue of whether cortical and

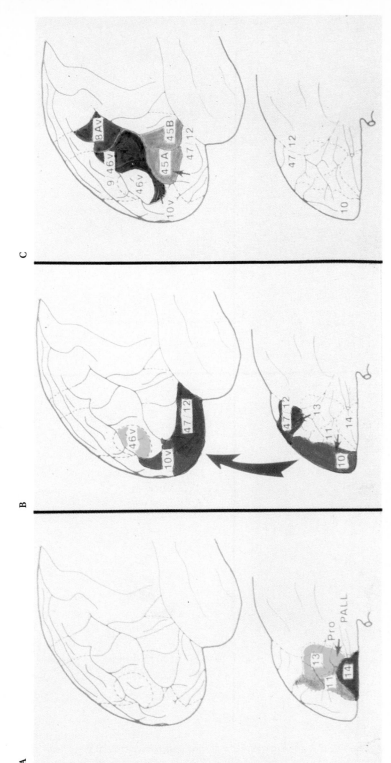

Fig. 9. Diagrams showing architectonic areas in the basoventral, or paleocortical, trend in the human prefrontal cortex arranged in stages within the orbital (A), orbital and ventrolateral (B), as well as caudolateral (C) regions (Petrides and Pandya, 1995)

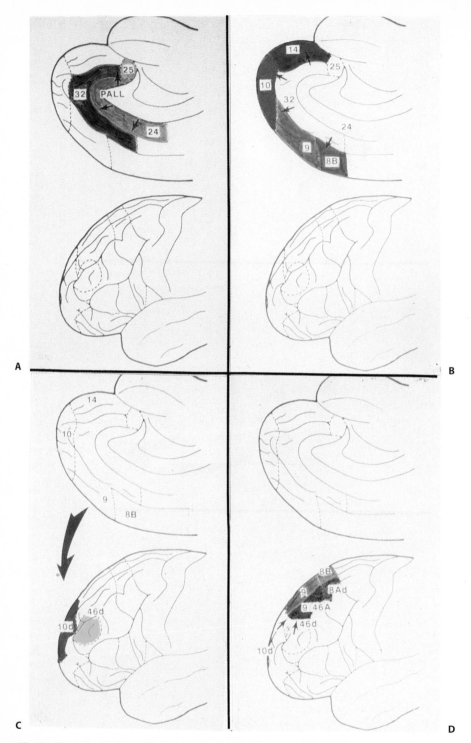

Fig. 10. Diagrams showing architectonic areas in the mediodorsal, or archicortical, trend in the human prefrontal cortex arranged in stages within the medial (**A, B**), rostrolateral (**C**), as well as caudolateral (**D**) regions (Petrides and Pandya, 1995)

subcortical connectivity reflects such organization. We will describe intrinsic connections, long association pathways, and finally the thalamic and striatal relationships of the prefrontal cortex in monkey. Because these connections have been
examined using classically defined architectonic areas, the following description is
based on the terminology used in previously published studies.

Connections of the Prefrontal Cortex

Intrinsic Connections

A given area of the prefrontal cortex projects in two directions to adjoining cortices (Barbas and Pandya 1989). In the paleocortical trend (Fig. 11A), the orbital
proisocortical area is related to surrounding areas 13, 12, 11 and 14. Area 13 in turn
projects back to the proisocortical area, as well as to areas 12, 11, and 14. Area 12
has efferents to areas 11, 13, and 14, as well as to the ventral portion of areas 10 and
46. Area 46 projects to areas 12 and 10 rostroventrally on the one hand, and to area
8 on the other. Area 8 in turn projects rostrally to area 46, to dorsal area 8, and
caudally to area 6. In the archicortical trend (Fig. 11B), medial proisocortical area
32 has efferents to areas 25 and 14 ventrally, to area 24 caudally, and to areas 9 and
10 dorsally. Area 9 in turn projects medially to proisocortical areas 32 and 24, and
laterally to dorsal area 10 and area 46. Area 46 has connections to areas 9 and 10,
and also to dorsal areas 8 and 6. Finally, dorsal area 8 projects rostrally to dorsal
area 46 and area 9, caudally to dorsal area 6, and to ventral area 8.

Thus, within the two architectonic trends of the prefrontal cortex, each area
seems to project to less differentiated areas on the one hand and to more differentiated areas on the other. Additionally, the predominant connections of a given
region are contained within its respective trend. It is important to note, however,
that there are interconnections between the two trends at certain levels, e.g.,
between areas 9 and 12, and between the dorsal and ventral portions of area 8
(Pandya and Barnes 1987).

Long Association Connections

Just as a given prefrontal area has a specific pattern of intrinsic connectivity, it also
is related to post-Rolandic regions in a systematic matter.

Somatosensory

The association areas of the parietal lobe are viewed as belonging to two
architectonic trends (Pandya and Seltzer 1982; Fig. 12A). Thus, the paleocortical
trend can be viewed as arising from the insular proisocortical and pericentral
opercular regions, passing through successive architectonic stages that culminate
in the cortices of the inferior parietal lobule (Fig. 6C). Similarly, the areas of the

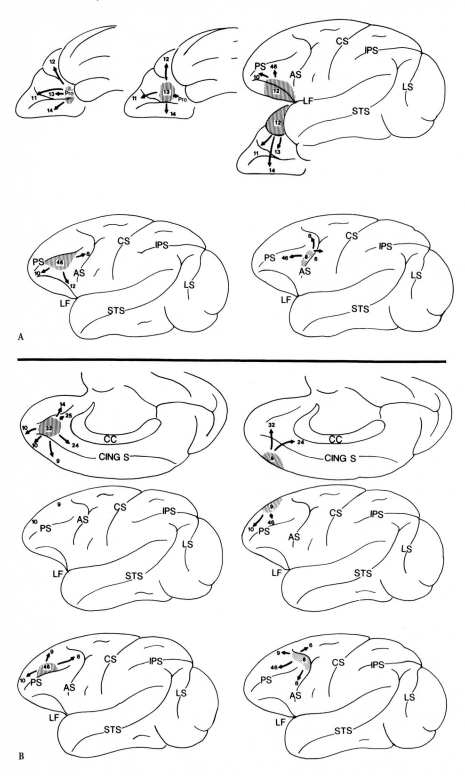

A

B

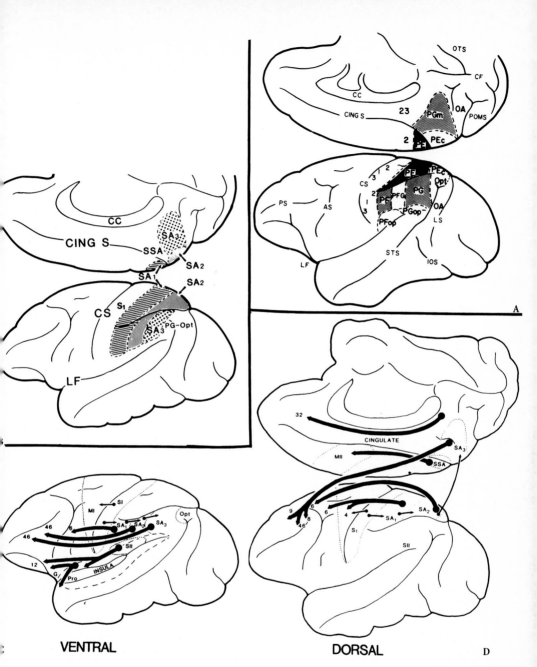

VENTRAL

DORSAL

D

Fig. 12. A Diagrams showing the architectonic parcellation of the posterior parietal cortex of the rhesus monkey (Pandya and Seltzer 1982). **B** Diagrammatic representations of the three subdivisions, SA1, SA2, SA3, of the association cortex of the inferior and superior parietal lobules. **C** Frontal lobe connections of the inferior parietal lobule (ventral or paleocortical trend). **D** Frontal lobe connections of the superior parietal lobule (dorsal or archicortical trend)

Fig. 11. Diagrams showing the intrinsic connections of the paleocortical (**A**) and archicortical (**B**) trends of the prefrontal cortex in the rhesus monkey

superior and medial parietal cortices are thought to have progressed from the archicortical moiety, and can be traced in successive steps through the proisocortical region of the cingulate gyrus (Fig. 6C), culminating in the subregions of the superior parietal lobule (Pandya and Yeterian 1985).

The cortex of the posterior parietal region has been divided into three broad sectors – first-order, SA1; second-order, SA2; and third-order, SA3, sensory association regions – from rostral to caudal within both the inferior (IPL) and superior (SPL) parietal lobules (Chavis and Pandya 1976; Fig. 12B). Each of these sectors has a different overall pattern of connectivity with the frontal cortex. Thus, within the inferior parietal region, SA1 (area PF) has connections to the ventral premotor cortex (area 6) and to the precentral and frontal opercula. SA2 of the IPL (rostral area PFG and the cortex of the lower lip of the intraparietal sulcus) projects to ventral area 46. Finally, SA3 of the IPL (rostral area PG and caudal area PFG) has efferents mainly to rostral area 46 in the lower bank of the principal sulcus (Fig. 12C). Likewise, within the superior parietal region, SA1 (area PE) projects to the caudal premotor cortex (dorsal area 6) and to the supplementary motor cortex (area MII). SA2 of the SPL (area PEc) has efferents to rostral premotor cortex (dorsal area 6), as well as to MII. SA3 on the medial parietal surface (area PGm) projects to the dorsal portions of area 8 and of areas 46 and 9 (Pandya and Yeterian 1990; Fig. 12D).

Thus, it appears that the regions of the IPL, which are tied to the face, head, and neck representations of ventral area SI, are connected to the ventral sector of the prefrontal cortex as well as to the gustatory area of the prefrontal operculum, whereas the regions of the SPL, which are related to the trunk and limb representations of dorsal area SI, project to the dorsal portion of the prefrontal cortex. This pattern of differential connectivity is consistent with the concept of a dual origin of the cerebral cortex in both the prefrontal and the parietal cortices.

Visual

Like the somatosensory system, the visual areas of the occipitotemporal cortex are proposed to have evolved from both proisocortical and archicortical moieties (Rosene and Pandya 1983). Two distinct trends can be traced, beginning in the proisocortex of the temporal pole (Pandya and Yeterian 1990). The paleocortical trend progresses ventrolaterally through the inferotemporal region (areas TE1, TE2, and TE3) to the association and primary visual areas (lateral areas OA, OB, and OC) of the occipital lobe (Fig. 13A). The archicortical trend is viewed as

Fig. 13. Diagrammatic representations of the distribution of different architectonic areas within the paleocortical trend (**A**) of the inferotemporal and lateral occipital regions, and the archicortical trend (**B**) in the paraphippocampal gyrus and medial, dorsal and ventral occipital areas, of the visual system of the rhesus monkey. **C** depicts visual association regions VA1, VA2 and VA3 of the inferotemporal cortex, and **D** shows their long association connections to the prefrontal cortex. **E** depicts long association connections to the frontal lobe from visual association areas on the medial, dorsal and ventral surfaces of the cerebral hemisphere

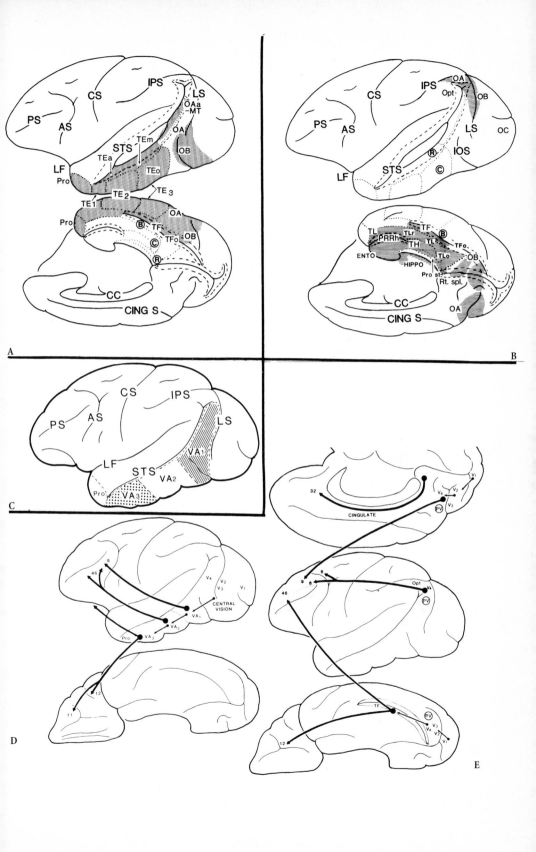

progressing ventromedially in successive steps through the posterior parahippocampal gyrus (areas TH, TL, TF, and the prostriate area) and occipital lobe regions (ventral and medial areas OA, OB, and OC; Fig. 13B).

The visual association areas of the ventrolateral occipital and inferotemporal cortices belonging to the paleocortical trend can be divided into three rostrocaudal sectors – first-order, VA1; second-order, VA2; and third-order, VA3, visual association regions (Chavis and Pandya 1976) (Fig. 13C). VA1 (lateral prestriate cortex and caudal area TE3) projects to area 8, whereas VA2 (rostral area TE3 and area TE2) has efferents mainly to area 46 but also to the rostral portion of area 8 below the level of the principal sulcus. VA3 (area TE1) has a distinctive connection to areas 12 and 11 (Pandya and Yeterian 1990; Fig. 13D).

Within the archicortical trend, the medial and dorsal prestriate area (dorsolateral area V4 and dorsomedial prestriate region) projects to dorsal area 8 and to area 9. The rostroventral peristriate belt area projects to area 46 within the upper bank of the principal sulcus, and to area 12 on the orbital surface (Pandya and Yeterian 1990; Fig. 13E).

Thus, the inferotemporal and lateral prestriate areas subserving central vision project preferentially to ventrolateral and orbital prefrontal regions. In contrast, the dorsolateral, medial, and ventromedial occipitotemporal cortices subserving peripheral vision project mainly to dorsal and medial prefrontal areas.

Auditory

The auditory association cortex of the superior temporal gyrus classically has been considered to be a single region. In recent years, however, it has been parcellated into a number of discrete areas having progressive architectonic differentiation: areas Pro and Ts1 rostrally having a relatively rudimentary laminar pattern, areas Ts2 and Ts3 more caudally, which show an intermediate pattern of architectonic differentiation, and areas paAlt and Tpt most caudally, which have the greatest degree of laminar differentiation (Pandya and Sanides 1973; Fig. 14B).

Like the somatosensory and visual association areas, the cortex of the superior temporal gyrus has been divided into first-order, AA1, second-order, AA2, and third-order, AA3, sectors (Chavis and Pandya 1976; Fig. 14A). Each of these sectors has been found to have a distinctive pattern of prefrontal connectivity. Thus, AA1 (areas Tpt and paAlt) projects mainly to dorsal area 8, whereas AA2 (areas Ts3 and Ts2) has efferents to the dorsal and ventral portions of area 46 as well as to areas 9 and 10. AA3 (areas Ts1 and Pro) projects to areas 12 and 13 on the orbital surface and to areas 25 and 32 on the medial surface of the frontal lobe (Pandya and Yeterian 1990; Fig. 14C).

It appears that highly differentiated areas of AA1 are connected with the caudal prefrontal region, which also is characterized by a high degree of laminar differentiation. In contrast, the relatively less differentiated areas of AA3 are related to orbital and medial prefrontal cortices with similar architectonic features. The areas of AA2, which appear to have an intermediate pattern of laminar differ-

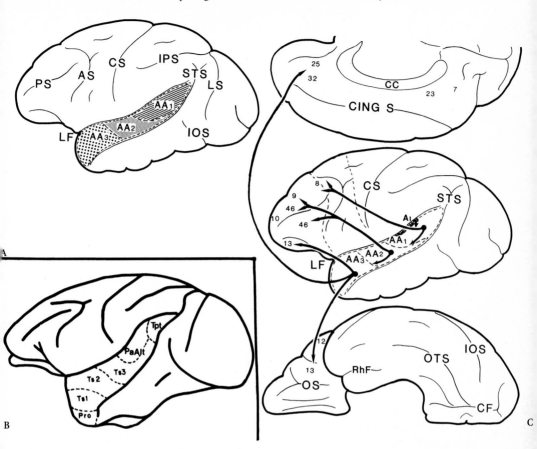

Fig. 14. A shows auditory association regions AA1, AA2, and AA3 of the superior temporal gyrus, and C depicts the connections of these regions to the prefrontal cortex. B shows the architectonic subdivisions of the superior temporal gyrus according to Pandya and Sanides (1973). Abbreviations: paAlt, lateral parakoniocortex; Pro, proisocortex; Tpt, temporoparietal cortex; Ts1, Ts2, Ts3, temporalis superior 1, 2, 3

entiation, project preferentially to lateral prefrontal cortices that have intermediate laminar characteristics. This pattern of connectivity, in which pre- and post-Rolandic areas having similar architectonic features are strongly interrelated via long association connections, seems also to characterize the prefrontal connectivity of somatosensory and visual association areas (Pandya and Yeterian 1985).

Paralimbic

The cortical zone that occupies a position between sensory association areas and limbic cortices has been termed the paralimbic region (e.g., Yeterian and Pandya 1988). This region, which contains several discrete cortical areas, is characterized

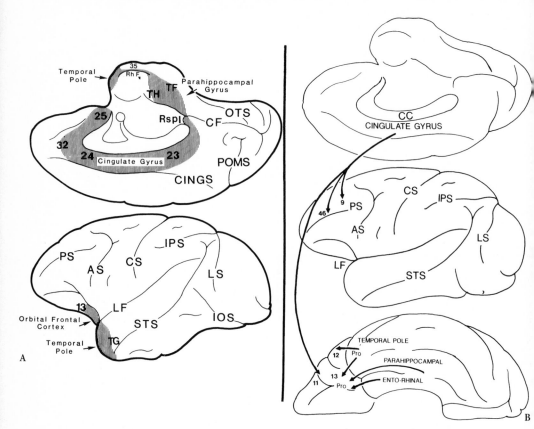

Fig. 15. A shows the various paralimbic areas in the medial and orbitofrontal cortices of the cerebral hemisphere in the rhesus monkey (Yeterian and Pandya 1988). Note the distribution of paralimbic areas on the orbital surface and the paleo-olfactory region (area 13); in the medial prefrontal cortex (areas 25 and 32); in the cingulate gyrus (areas 24, 23, and the retrosplenial area, Rspl); in the parahippocampal gyrus (areas TH and TF); in the perirhinal cortex (area 35); and in the temporal pole (area TG or 38). **B** depicts the frontal lobe connections from dorsal (cingulate, or archicortical) and ventral (temporal polar-parahippocampal, or paleocortical) paralimbic regions

by a predominance of infragranular layers and a weak or absent layer IV. Areas belonging to this category include the cingulate cortices (areas 32, 25, 24, and 23), the temporal pole (area Pro), and the parahippocampal gyrus (areas TF and TH), as well as the caudal orbital frontal cortex (areas 13 and Pro; Fig. 15A).

There are differential connectional relationships between various paralimbic areas and the prefrontal cortex. The temporal polar region and the parahippocampal gyrus project strongly to the orbital frontal cortex, areas 12, 13, and orbital proisocortex. The cingulate gyrus is known to project predominantly to the lateral prefrontal region, area 9 and dorsal area 46, as well as to area 11 of the orbital frontal cortex. With regard to the two architectonic trends within the cerebral cortex, a differential pattern of prefrontal connectivity from paralimbic regions is not as clear as for the sensory association cortices. Nevertheless, the temporal proisocortex, which is part of the paleocortical trend, is related mainly to the orbital frontal cortex. In contrast, the cingulate gyrus, which belongs to the archicortical trend, projects predominantly to the dorsal prefrontal cortex. Thus, the connections of paralimbic cortices appear to be organized in a manner consistent with the concept of dual architectonic trends.

Multimodal

A number of post-Rolandic cortical regions have been designated as multimodal in nature on the basis of connectional and physiological investigations. The principal region is in the parietotemporal cortex, and consists of the upper bank of the superior temporal sulcus (STS; Fig. 16A) and the caudalmost portion of the inferior parietal lobule. Like the sensory association areas, the cortex of the upper bank of STS has been shown to contain a number of rostrocaudal subdivisions with differential architectonic and connectional features (Seltzer and Pandya 1989). With regard to prefrontal connectivity, the rostralmost division projects preferentially to the orbital and medial prefrontal cortices, whereas the caudalmost portion is related strongly to the caudal prefrontal region. The middle division of the cortex of the upper bank of STS projects mainly to the intermediate, dorsolateral portion of the prefrontal cortex (Fig. 16B). The parietal lobe multimodal area PG-Opt is connected mainly with prefrontal area 8 as well as with area 6. Thus, the subareas of the multimodal region of STS are related connectionally to prefrontal regions in a manner similar to post-Rolandic sensory association areas.

Subcortical

The concept of dual architectonic trends within the prefrontal cortex is consistent with the pattern of thalamic connectivity (e.g., Giguere and Goldman-Rakic 1988;

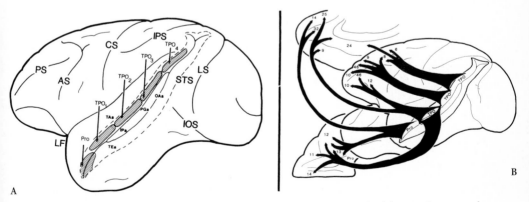

Fig. 16. A shows the subregions of the multimodal cortex of the upper bank of the superior temporal sulcus in the rhesus monkey, and **B** depicts the prefrontal connections of these areas

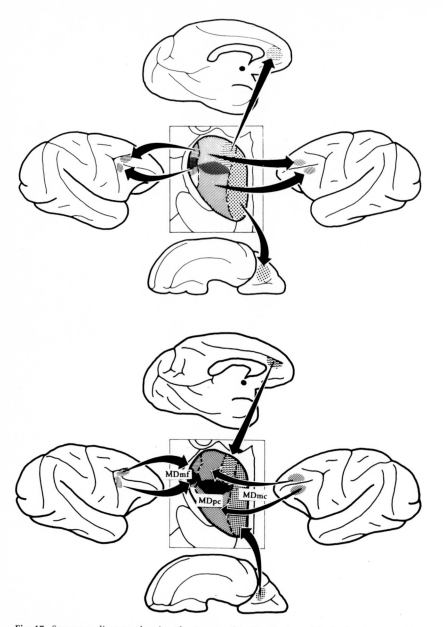

Fig. 17. Summary diagram showing the topographic distribution of both the thalamocortical and corticothalamic connections between the prefrontal cortex and the mediodorsal nucleus in the rhesus monkey (Siwek and Pandya 1991)

Siwek and Pandya 1991). As one progresses from less differentiated toward more highly elaborated prefrontal regions within each trend, there is a corresponding shift in connectivity from medial to lateral thalamic regions. Thus, the medial and orbital frontal proisocortical areas are related to the most medial portion of the

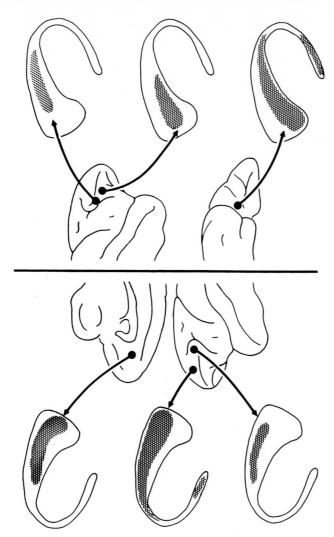

Fig. 18. Summary diagrams showing the connectional relationships between the dorsal or archicortical and ventral or paleocortical architectonic trends of the prefrontal cortex and the caudate nucleus in the sagittal plane in the rhesus monkey (Yeterian and Pandya 1991)

mediodorsal(MD) nucleus (magnocellular division, MDmc). The lateral prefrontal region is connected with the middle portion of the MD nucleus (parvocellular division, MDpc). Area 8, in contrast, is related to the lateral sector of the MD nucleus (multiform division, MDmf). Moreover, the paleocortical areas are related to ventral portions of the MD nucleus, whereas archicortical areas are connected strongly with dorsal portions. Therefore, the paleo- and archicortical trends have different overall patterns of connectivity with the MD nucleus (Fig. 17).

Corticostriatal connections of the prefrontal cortex also are organized in a manner consistent with dual architectonic trends (Yeterian and Pandya 1991). Areas belonging to the paleocortical trend project mainly to ventral portions of the head of the caudate nucleus, whereas those in the archicortical trend project strongly to the dorsal portions (Fig. 18). Within each trend, areas having relatively less laminar differentiation project mainly to the medial portion of the head of the caudate nucleus. In contrast, highly differentiated regions are connected mainly with lateral portions of the head of the caudate nucleus, whereas prefrontal areas having intermediate laminar characteristics are related to central portions.

Discussion

Beginning in the nineteenth century, many investigators proposed different theories of frontal lobe function (e.g., Ferrier 1876; Bianchi 1895; Jacobsen 1935; Nauta 1971; Teuber 1972; Luria 1973; Stuss and Benson 1986; Goldman-Rakic 1987; Fuster 1989; Shallice and Burgess 1991; Damasio and Anderson 1993). However, the precise manner in which the frontal lobe contributes to behavior is not fully understood. With the continuing development of brain imaging as well as molecular biological techniques, it is likely that we will attain a much more complete knowledge of the operations of the frontal lobe. Nevertheless, in the light of available data, it is possible to interrelate cellular and connectional features of the prefrontal cortex with different aspects of function, admittedly at a relatively gross morphological level.

Architectonics and Intrinsic Connections

At the architectonic level, the frontal lobe displays a systematic pattern of laminar organization, from relatively simple and undifferentiated cortices toward highly elaborated areas. Such progressions seem to arise from two basic moieties, one medial and the other ventral in location, with both culminating in the caudolateral portions of the prefrontal cortex. It is not unreasonable to assume that such architectonic progression may be associated with functional differentiation involving different prefrontal areas. A common problem for all organisms is making appropriate and withholding inappropriate responses under changing circum-

Frontal Lobe and the Cognitive Foundation of Behavioral Action

J.M. Fuster

Summary

Motor representations are hierarchically organized in dorsolateral frontal cortex. The highest, most global plans and schemes of action appear to be represented in prefrontal cortex, intermediate ones in premotor cortex, and the most elementary motor acts in primary motor cortex. The confluence of external and internal inputs on frontal cortex leads to the activation of frontal neuron networks representing different categories of action. The activation of these networks is the physiological substrate for the initiation and execution of behavioral action.

Sequences of deliberate action require the coordinated interplay of all stages of the frontal hierarchy. Two cognitive functions for temporal integration operate at every stage: active short-term memory and preparatory set. Both are most apparent and can best be studied in the prefrontal cortex, where the longest action sequences are represented and coordinated and where cross-temporal contingencies are mediated. The prefrontal cortex, in cooperation with subcortical and posterior cortical areas, ensures the retention of sensory information for prospective action and the preparatory set of motor systems for its execution. Both of these functions of the prefrontal cortex have been substantiated by neuropsychology, reversible lesion and microelectrode recording in the monkey, and neuroimaging in the human.

Introduction

The cortex of the frontal lobe is "motor cortex" in the broadest sense of the term. It is cortex essentially devoted to the representation and execution of a wide range of actions, from skeletal and ocular movements to speech, even perhaps to the "internal actions" of logical reasoning. The motor, executive character of the frontal lobe is an old idea, probably first expressed by Betz (1874), the Russian neuroanatomist, who simply extrapolated to the cerebral cortex a basic principle of neural organization that prevails at lower levels of the nerve axis, beginning with

Department of Psychiatry and Brain Research Institute, School of Medicine, University of California, 760 Westwood Plaza, Los Angeles, CA 90024, USA

A.R. Damasio et al. (Eds.)
Neurobiology of Decision-Making
© Springer-Verlag Berlin Heidelberg 1996

the spinal cord. The posterior moiety of the axis is largely allocated to sensory structures and functions, the anterior moiety to motor structures and functions. Of course, there are a few exceptions – notably the cerebellum – that result from the vicissitudes of neuroontogeny and that challenge the validity of that simplification, but by and large both basic and clinical neurosciences uphold the dichotomy.

The "motor" functions of the frontal cortex, however, can hardly be understood without considering that a large expanse of it, the cortex of association of the frontal lobe or prefrontal cortex, harbors a number of cognitive and emotional functions that may appear independent from motor function, yet provide it with essential support. More specifically, the cortex of the dorsolateral frontal convexity provides the cognitive substrate of motor action by sustaining such functions as memory and set that are indispensable for the organization of any complex, novel and deliberate behavior. The cortex of medial and inferior (orbital) frontal regions, on the other hand, sustains emotional and affective functions that critically determine or modulate social behavior. None of these structures and functions can be compartmentalized without danger of slipping into neophrenology. Further, it makes no sense to consider frontal cortex as a functional entity that is independent from posterior cortex and subcortical structures, with which it works in close cooperation. Nonetheless here, for heuristic reasons, I shall focus on the cognitive functions of dorsolateral frontal cortex as they pertain to behavioral action and to the topic of this conference.

Frontal Cortex in the Representation of Action

Every domain of action – e.g., skeletal movement, eye movement, speech – has its regional representation in dorsolateral frontal cortex. The region of representation includes parts of the three major subdivisions of that cortex: primary motor cortex, premotor cortex (including supplementary motor area; SMA), and prefrontal cortex. The three subdivisions are organized hierarchically, and so are the actions they represent within each action domain. Indeed, motor memory, like perceptual memory, is hierarchically organized (the subject is reviewed at length in Fuster 1994). It is an organization that reflects to some extent the ontogenetic order of frontal development, at least with regard to one criterion, namely, the order of myelination of the intrinsic and extrinsic connection fibers of the cortex of the frontal lobe. That cortical myelination order was first established by Flechsig (1901) at the turn of the century (Fig. 1).

The broadest schemes or plans of action are probably represented in the prefrontal cortex, which is the highest level of the frontal cortical hierarchy. Monkeys and humans with large dorsolateral prefrontal lesions cannot execute, presumably because they cannot represent, large schemes of action. Of course, when the schemes are extensive in the time domain, the subjects have trouble executing them also for another reason, that is, the inability to organize action in time (see

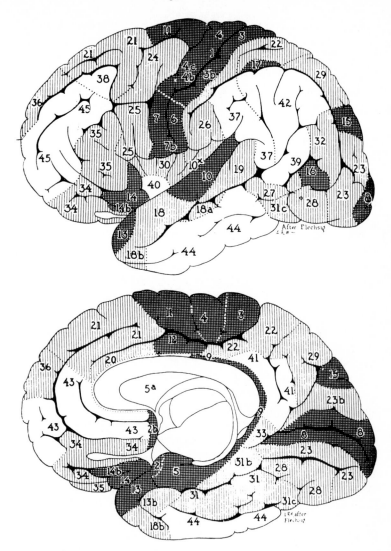

Fig. 1. Myelination order of cortical areas according to Flechsig (1901)

below). The fact remains, however, that motor representation at its highest level is impaired.

Just below the prefrontal cortex, the premotor areas seem to contain somewhat more concrete motor representations, schemes of action that are already defined by such parameters as spatial trajectory of movement, order of execution if relatively simple, and goal if relatively close in space and time. This stage includes the dorsal and medial SMA; there is no convincing neurophysiological evidence to conclude that this area has representational properties different from those of the rest of area 6 (Brodmann), although differences in somatotopy cannot be excluded.

The motor cortex of area 4 is the lowest stage of the frontal hierarchy for the representation of movement. There, imminent action is represented in its most concrete and specific terms. The neuronal populations of area 4 represent in their ensembles the vectors of action, in terms of direction and muscle groups, that the animal is about to execute (Georgopoulos et al. 1986).

The frontal cortex is not the only store of motor memory. There are now good reasons to suspect that, once established, reflex and automatic acts – in other words, much of what has been termed "procedural memory" – are represented outside the neocortex, especially in the basal ganglia and the cerebellum (Thompson 1986; Alexander and Crutcher 1990b). There is one important, albeit teleological, reason why this is probably so: to free the frontal cortex for the representation and execution of novel deliberate actions.

Nowhere is the frontal hierarchy of representation more evident than in the highest primate and in the highest action domain: the spoken language. The most complex, conceptual, and extended forms of speech are probably represented, before they are executed, in dorsolateral prefrontal cortex. Clinical neuro-psychology provides the most convincing evidence that this is the case. Indeed there is a prefrontal aphasia. The speech of the patient with extensive lesion of dorsolateral prefrontal cortex is characterized by generally impoverished linguis-tic structure, as if the patient had lost the ability to "propositionise" (Jackson 1915). His speech production is low and lacks fluidity, generally being made up of short sentences that mostly express commonplace information and with few de-pendent clauses (Lhermitte et al. 1972; Albert et al. 1981). As is the case with most aphasias, the prefrontal aphasia is especially severe when the lesion affects the left or dominant hemisphere.

Lesions that affect premotor cortex, including SMA, can also induce an apha-sia with properties similar to those of the prefrontal aphasia, but more severe. The speech of some patients with premotor injury not only has the characteristics noted above for the prefrontal disorder but, in addition, tends to be halting and monotonal (Luria 1970; Goldberg et al. 1981). The deficit becomes dramatic when the affected cortex is that of the inferior frontal convolution on the left side (Broca's area). Broca's aphasia, with its well-known agrammatism, telegraphic style, and almost nonexistent syntax, reveals the breakdown of primitive and essential representations at the lowest level of the speech hierarchy of the frontal lobe. Below that level there is still the primary motor cortex, where the motility of the oropharingeal apparatus is represented. Of course, lesion there can also affect speech, but only for lack of effector function.

In summary, then, the hierarchical organization of speech representations in frontal cortex epitomizes the hierarchical organization of frontal memory in all domains of action. Larger behavioral structures, in space and time, seem repre-sented in prefrontal cortex, intermediate ones in premotor cortex, and the smallest ones in motor cortex.

Frontal Cortex in the Initiation of Action

Almost constantly in the awake state, under the influence of internal drives and external stimuli, new and old schemes of action (mental action or behavioral action) are formed and activated, or reactivated, presumably in the neuronal networks of frontal cortex. Once the action scheme has been formed, and if the circumstances are favorable, the individual may decide to act. What leads to the decision to act, and to act in a certain way? The question in almost inextricable from the argument about free will. It has been the subject of long and heated debate by philosophers, jurists, psychologists, and neuroscientists. It is an issue that is complicated by questions about conscious deliberation that for now remain unresolved at any level of discourse.

From the point of view of today's neuroscience, however, two facts appear increasingly clear: 1) there is no such thing as a neural "center of will," in the frontal lobe or anywhere else; and 2) the cortex of the frontal lobe is the ultimate "common path" for the enactment of all deliberate decisions. Let us briefly consider the reasons.

Any pretense to ascribe the origin of willed action to a sector of the frontal lobe (e.g., prefrontal cortex, SMA) ignores the overwhelming evidence that, probably anywhere in it, neurons are constantly under a barrage of neural influences from many sectors of the rest of the nervous system. Indeed, the frontal cortex, especially the prefrontal neocortex, is the best connected of all cortical regions (Fuster 1989). Afferent fibers arrive to it from the brain stem, the diencephalon, the limbic system, both amygdala and hippocampus, and other cortical regions (Fig. 2). The latter bring to the prefrontal cortex profuse inputs from extensive and numerous areas of sensory processing and perceptual memory in postrolandic cortex. In this context, it is inconceivable that the decision to implement a course of action should originate autonomously, de novo, in frontal cortex.

More plausible is the notion that the decision to act, like the formulation of the plan, is the result of the competition between diverse, sometimes conflicting, neural influences converging on prefrontal cortex. That decision, as well as the general course of action, would be the resulting "vector" from that competition of influences. Thereafter, the particulars of the action would be determined by the principles of cognitive operation and organization of action discussed in the next section. Whether the competing influences enter conscious awareness or not would mark the difference between "determinism" and "free will," at least as perceived by the acting subject. By this reasoning, the concept of a "center of will" anywhere in the brain is both superfluous and misleading.

Once the decision to act has been made, the representational networks of the frontal cortex become operational. Action cannot be separated from motor memory, because the same networks that represent the action at any level of abstraction now become the agents. First the prefrontal networks are recruited, where action in its most abstract form – the scheme, the plan – is represented. Then the enactment involves progressively lower stages of the frontal motor hierarchy, that is, the premotor cortex and, ultimately, the motor cortex, where the

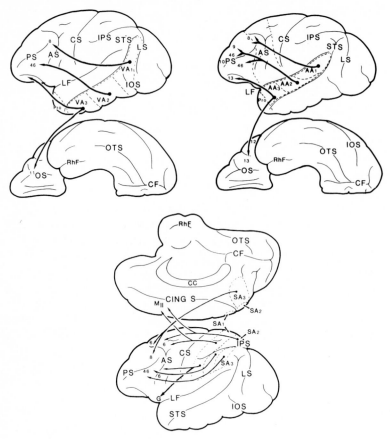

Fig. 2. Afferent connections to prefrontal cortex from other cortical areas, according to Pandya and Yeterian (1985)

"microgenesis of the action" (Brown 1987) takes place. Two important caveats are necessary here. First, the processing is not all serial, successive, from the top down; there is abundant parallel processing down the hierarchy, as well as serial, and many recurrent loops are involved in that processing. Second, some of those recurrent loops are extracortical; they course through subcortical structures, notably the basal ganglia and the lateral thalamus (Alexander and Crutcher 1990a).

Just before behavioral action is initiated, a surface-negative potential wave can be recorded over the frontal lobe, even on the intact scalp; the wave originates over prefrontal cortex, progresses over premotor cortex, and eventually terminates in the vertex region, over primary motor cortex. The anterior and earliest component of that wave is called the "contingent negative variation" (CNV), whereas the posterior and later component is called the Bereitschaftspotential or "readiness potential" (Walter et al. 1964; Kornhuber and Deecke 1965; Brunia et al. 1985). That negative wave, as a whole, reflects the underlying and progressive recruit-

ment of neuronal networks of the frontal motor hierarchy involved in the processing of the action, beginning with prefrontal cortex and ending up in motor cortex.
Curiously, the onset of the wave seems to precede the conscious awareness of the
intention to move (Libet 1985).

Frontal Cortex in the Organization of Action

The execution of an extended sequence of behavioral actions toward a goal cannot
be understood without postulating, in addition to the hierarchical processing
briefly outlined above, the continued and precise interaction between sensory
inputs and motor outputs at a high level of the motor hierarchy. To understand the
mechanisms of this interaction, it is necessary to envision a place for the cortex of
the frontal lobe in what has been termed the perception-action cycle (Fuster 1989).
This is a basic biological principle of operation of all organisms in their environment (Weizsäcker 1950). It consists of the circular cybernetic interaction between
the two, organism and environment, depicted schematically in Figure 3. Sensory
input leads to motor output, which leads to change in the environment, which
leads to feedback to the senses, which leads to new sensory input, and so on.

Whenever in a complex and novel sequence, sensory input and motor output
are separated by time, then the prefrontal cortex, which we postulate at the top of
the perception-action cycle (Fig. 4), must intervene to close the gap and to mediate
the contingency between sensation and movement. It does so by two complemen-

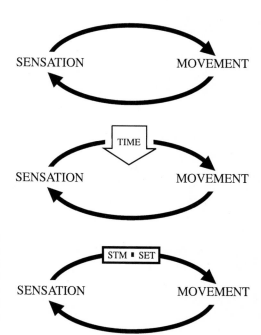

Fig. 3. Scheme of the perception-action
cycle. In the middle diagram, interruption
of the cycle by a time span. Bottom, time is
bridged by two temporally integrative
functions of frontal cortex: active short-
term memory (STM) and preparatory set
(SET). (See text under Frontal Cortex in
the Organization of Action.)

SENSORY
HIERARCHY

MOTOR
HIERARCHY

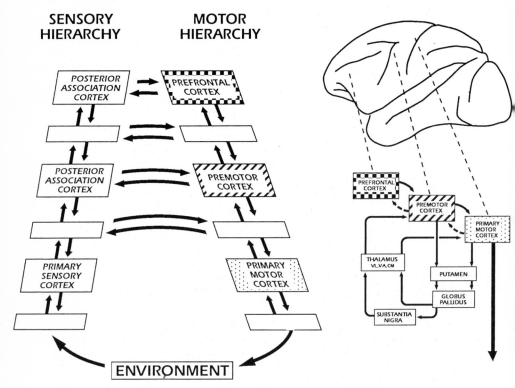

Fig. 4. Functional anatomy of the cortex in the perception-action cycle. Blank rectangles denote subareas or intermediate areas. All arrows denote anatomically identified connections. Al right, frontal-subcortical motor processing loops

tary time-bridging functions in which the dorsolateral prefrontal cortex is most critically involved. One is a temporally "retrospective" function of short-term memory, the other a temporally "prospective" function of preparatory motor set. These two functions are the basis for the critical role of the prefrontal cortex in the temporal organization of behavior, in the syntax of the action to use Lashley's (1951) term. I devote the rest of this chapter to summarizing some evidence for these two cognitive functions of the prefrontal cortex in monkey and man. The evidence comes from three sources: neuropsychology, neurophysiology, and neuroimaging.

Active Short-Term Memory

The dorsolateral prefrontal cortex of the primate plays a critical role in the temporary retention of any given memory in active state. That memory may be old or new; in either case, it is most likely represented by a widely distributed network that extends beyond prefrontal cortex. This cortex is essential, however, to hold that entire network in the active state. Insofar as the memory is needed for pro-spective action, say in performance of a task, the activated memory coincides with what has been characterized as "working memory." The concept of active memory, however, transcends that of "working memory" because it includes conscious remembering. Thus, active memory is a concept better suited to the phenomenol-ogy of human memory (Fuster 1994).

A characteristic manifestation of the human prefrontal syndrome is the deficit in recent memory (Stuss and Benson 1986). The patient has difficulty remember-ing recent events, though long-term memory appears to remain intact. On close analysis, however, it frequently becomes obvious that the memory deficit is com-plicated by troubles in general drive and attention which may, by themselves, account for the apparent trouble in retention inasmuch as they interfere with the acquisition of memory in the first place (Luria 1966; Barbizet 1970). For good reason it has been said that the frontal patient can remember but "forgets to remember" (Hécaen and Albert 1978).

Nevertheless, formal neuropsychological testing has now firmly demonstrated that the patient with substantial dorsolateral lesion suffers from a short-term memory deficit that is irreducible to impairment in any other psychological func-tion. This deficit is supramodal, that is, affects memoranda of all sensory modalities, and becomes especially evident through working-memory tests, such as delay tasks (Lewinsohn 1972; Milner et al. 1985; Freedman and Oscar-Berman 1986).

It was in the monkey, however, that the delay-task deficit from dorsolateral prefrontal lesion was first demonstrated (Jacobsen 1935) and later extensively confirmed. Reversible cryogenic lesions, which allow the fine control of certain task parameters (e.g., length of delay) and the use of each animal repeatedly as its own control, has permitted us to ascertain that the functional depression of dorsolateral prefrontal cortex induces deficits in active memory for sensory infor-mation of the visual (Bauer and Fuster 1976), auditory (Sierra-Paredes and Fuster 1993), and tactile (Shindy et al. 1994) modalities.

By microelectrode recording from monkeys performing delay tasks, the neuronal correlates of active short-term memory have been revealed (Fuster and Alexander 1971; Fuster 1973; Niki 1974; Funahashi et al. 1989). We now know that neurons in the area of the sulcus principalis undergo elevated sustained firing during the memorization of sensory stimuli that the monkey must retain for actions it must perform in the short term. Clearly, the elevated firing of prefrontal cells reflects the activation of prefrontal networks in charge of maintaining sensory memory for that short term. A note of caution is needed here, however; the dorsolateral prefrontal cortex does not perform its memory function all by itself but in close cooperation with other neocortical areas, notably the association areas of posterior cortex (e.g., the inferotemporal cortex if the memory is visual; Fuster et al. 1985). Thus, whereas it is correct to conclude that the dorsolateral prefrontal cortex is essential for active short-term memory toward action, it is erroneous to claim that this cortex is the repository, let alone the center, of active or working memory. Active memory is a global cortical function, however essential a prefrontal territory of cortex may be for it when the memory serves behavioral action.

The sustained excitation of prefrontal cells during active short-term memory has its metabolic expression in the neuroimage of the human performing a delay task. Dorsolateral prefrontal metabolism or blood flow has been seen to increase during performance of spatial delay tasks (Jonides et al. 1993). We have seen it in a non-spatial visual delay task (Swartz et al. 1995). In our study, 18 subjects were trained to perform a delayed matching to sample task with visual stimuli that consisted of abstract images which the subject had to memorize in each trial for a few seconds (Fig. 5). A task with the same stimuli and demanding the same motor responses, but without the memory requirement, was used for control purposes. The subjects were requested to perform the two tasks after injection and during central uptake of isotopically marked fluordeoxyglucose. By subtracting the levels of glucose uptake during the memory task from those during the control task, it became apparent that the former task induced relatively high activation of certain cortical areas, among them most notably the dorsolateral prefrontal cortex (Fig. 6). In conclusion, neuroimaging studies confirm at a macro scale what microelectrode studies led us to believe: that the neuronal networks of dorsolateral prefrontal cortex are exceptionally active during active memory.

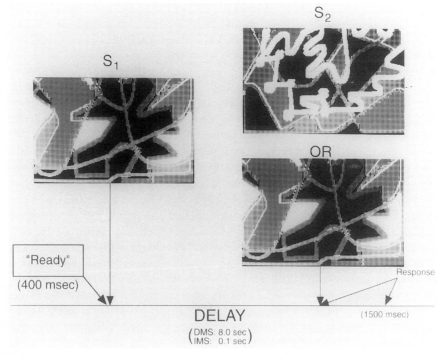

Fig. 5. Schematic diagram of delayed matching to sample task with abstract pictures. Control task is identical, but without a memory requirement (8-sec delay). The subject's response is the pressing of a button with one hand for match and another button with the other hand for mismatch

Fig. 6. Areas marked by shading (solid black or pattern) are relatively more activated during the memory task (Fig. 5) than during the control task

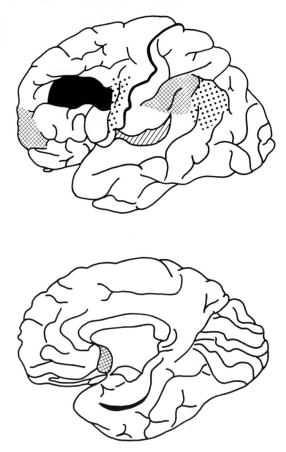

Preparatory Set

Whereas the memory deficit of the frontal-lobe patient has often been a matter of controversy, there has always been general agreement on the patient's impaired ability to make plans and to execute them. Indeed, the difficulty in planning and preparing for future action is probably the most characteristic feature of the dorsolateral prefrontal syndrome. Much of that difficulty is undoubtedly based on the absence of a suitable neural substrate for the representation of future action, a deficit in what Ingvar (1985) termed the "memory of the future." Some of the trouble, however, can be attributed to an impairment in the ability to prepare, to set, the motor apparatus for prospective action.

This ability to set motor systems for action is most likely distributed throughout the dorsolateral frontal cortex. Its electrophysiological correlates can be recognized at all levels of the frontal motor hierarchy, i.e., prefrontal, premotor, and motor. In all probability, neurons active in the motor setting contribute to the CNV and the "readiness potential." Nowhere, however, are the frontal neuron contributions to preparatory set more evident than at the level of the single unit.

When a monkey is getting ready to execute as motor act, as during the delay of a delay task, a series of firing changes can be observed in the discharge of frontal cells. One is the sustained elevated discharge of prefrontal neurons that I have attributed to short-term memory. Here I will add that this discharge, as might be expected of a short-term memory phenomenon, tends to decrease as the period of delay progresses. In addition to those "memory cells," and intermingled with them, one can find cells that show the converse phenomenon, a gradual increase in firing as the response grows near. Whereas the memory cells seem to look back in time to the cue or whatever the monkey must remember, these "set cells" seem to look forward in time to the forthcoming motor response.

"Set cells" can be found anywhere in lateral frontal cortex. The notion that they are indeed involved motor set is supported by two empirical facts: 1) the time differences with which, before the motor act, they come into play in different frontal regions, and 2) the relationship between their discharge and the probability (i.e., predictability) of the act, at least in some of its particulars.

Before the motor act, prefrontal "set cells" are the first to accelerate their firing. Given enough time between a cuing stimulus and the response it calls for, these cells are seen to anticipate the response by 10 sec or more (Fuster et al. 1982). "Set cells" in premotor cortex anticipate the response by 2 to 3 sec at most (DiPellegrino and Wise 1991). Those with the shortest lead-time are the cells of motor cortex, which anticipate the movement at most by a few hundreds of milliseconds (Tanji and Evarts 1976). Thus, in the preparation for the motor act, there seems to be a temporal gradient of recruitment of frontal cells, from the highest to the lowest levels of the motor hierarchy.

That temporal gradient appears to correspond to the order of complexity of motor representations in frontal cortices as postulated above, with the scheme of the action on top, in prefrontal cortex, and its most concrete aspects at the bottom, in motor cortex. Thus, it is reasonable to infer that the order of recruitment of cells from the highest to the lowest frontal stage reflects the progressive activation of their motor representation networks as the action develops.

However, because no action has yet occurred while these neuronal changes happen, it is also reasonable to infer that the activation of any given frontal network has the objective of priming structures below for the actions anticipated. The lower in the hierarchy the structure is, and the more concrete and less imminent the action its networks represent, the later these networks are activated to ready the stages below. Thus, prefrontal networks, which represent the most global aspects of action, would come in first to set premotor networks representing more concrete acts, and the next premotor networks would do the same with motor networks under them. The temporal gradient of cellular recruitment would thus reflect the order in which frontal representational networks become operational.

Further evidence that prefrontal networks engage in preparatory set has come from a study in which we made the concrete aspects of a forthcoming motor response more or less certain for the animal (Quintana and Fuster 1992). The task was a delay task in which the cue, a color, connoted with different degrees of probability the direction of a manual response a few seconds later. Under these

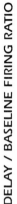

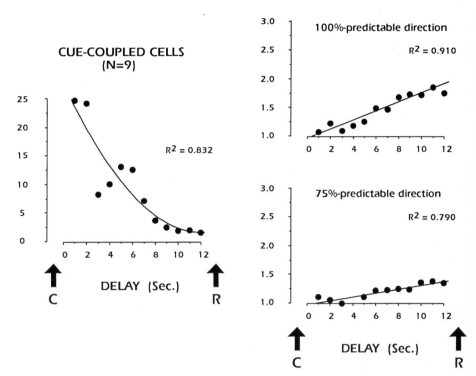

Fig. 7. Discharge of sensory-coupled (left) and motor-coupled (right) prefrontal units during the delay period of a double-contingency delay task. In it, the direction of a manual response at the end of a delay is determined by the combination of two separate cues, one at the beginning and the other at the end of the delay. As a result, if the first cue (C) is of a given color, the monkey can predict with 100% certainty the direction of the response; if C is of some other color, the animal can predict the response with only 75% certainty. Note the temporal descent of firing in sensory-coupled units ("memory cells") and acceleration in motor-coupled units ("set cells"). Note also the steeper firing increase of motor-coupled cells when the monkey can predict with 100% (vs 75%) probability of success the direction of the impending motor response

conditions we observed that the accelerating prefrontal cell discharge in anticipation of motor response was proportional to the predictability of the direction of that response (Fig. 7).

Finally, evidence of frontal cortex involvement in motor set comes from our imaging study in the human (Swartz et al. 1995). During performance of the delayed visual matching task, more activation was observed in dorsolateral prefrontal cortex, and downstream in premotor and motor cortex, than during the control task. In view of the fact that in both tasks the subject was exposed to the same number of visual stimuli and had to perform the same number of motor responses, the difference in frontal activations between the two tasks can only be explained by differences in "duty cycle:" during the task with delay between stimulus and response, the subject spent more time memorizing and preparing to respond than during the control, non-memory, task (even though the preparation was for a hand response, unspecified until the second stimulus appeared for the choice of hand). Arguably, the prefrontal activation might be due only or mainly to memory (see above, Active Short-term Memory), but the activations of premotor and motor cortices must have been due to the involvement of these cortices in preparatory set.

In conclusion, both microelectrode and neuroimaging data provide compelling evidence for the role of frontal cortex in preparatory set, one of the cognitive functions deemed essential for the temporal organization of behavior. Only further research can elucidate the underlying neural mechanisms.

Acknowledgments. The research by the author reported in this article was supported by grants from the National Institute of Mental Health, the National Science Foundation, and the Office of Naval Research.

References

Albert ML, Goodglass H, Helm NA, Rubens AB, Alexander MP (1981) Clinical aspects of dysphasia. New York, Springer

Alexander GE, Crutcher MD (1990a) Functional architecture of basal ganglia circuits: neural substrates of parallel processing. Trends Neurosci 13:266–271

Alexander GE, Crutcher MD (1990b) Preparation for movement: Neural representations of intended direction in three motor areas of the monkey. J Neurophysiol 64:133–150

Barbizet J (1970) Human Memory and its pathology. San Francisco, Freeman

Bauer RH, Fuster JM (1976) Delayed-matching and delayed-response deficit from cooling dorsolateral prefrontal cortex in monkeys. J Comp Physiol Psychol 90:293–302

Betz W (1874) Anatomischer Nachweis zweier Gehirncentra. Centralblatt für die medizinische Wissenschaften 12:578–580, 595–559

Brown JW (1987) The microstructure of action. In: Perecman E (ed) The frontal lobes revisited. New York, IRBN Press, pp 250–272

Brunia CHM, Haagh SAVM, Scheirs JGM (1985) Waiting to respond: Electrophysiological measurements in man during preparation for a voluntary movement. In: Heuer H, Kleinbeck U, Schmidt K-H (eds) Motor behavior. New York, Springer

Di Pellegrino G, Wise SP (1991) A neurophysiological comparison of three distinct regions of the primate frontal lobe. Brain 114:951–978

Flechsig P (1901) Developmental (myelogenetic) localisation of the cerebral cortex in the human subject. Lancet 2:1027–1029

Freedman M, Oscar-Berman M (1986) Bilateral frontal lobe disease and selective delayed response deficits in humans. Behav Neurosci 100:337–342

Funahashi S, Bruce CJ, Goldman-Rakic PS (1989) Mnemonic coding of visual space in the monkey's dorsolateral prefrontal cortex. J Neurophysiol 61:331–349

Fuster JM (1973) Unit activity in prefrontal cortex during delayed-response performance: Neuronal correlates of transient memory. J Neurophysiol 36:61–78

Fuster JM (1989) The prefrontal cortex: anatomy, physiology, and neuropsychology of the frontal lobe. New York, Raven

Fuster JM (1994) Memory in the cerebral cortex: An empirical approach to neural networks in the human and nonhuman primate. Cambridge, MIT Press

Fuster JM, Alexander GE (1971) Neuron activity related to short-term memory. Science 173:652–654

Fuster JM, Bauer RH, Jervey JP (1982) Cellular discharge in the dorsolateral prefrontal cortex of the monkey in cognitive tasks. Exp Neurol 77:679–694

Fuster JM, Bauer RH, Jervey JP (1985) Functional interactions between inferotemporal and prefrontal cortex in a cognitive task. Brain Res 330:299–307

Georgopoulos AP, Schwartz AB, Kettner RE (1986) Neuronal population coding of movement direction. Science 233:1416–1419

Goldberg G, Mayer NH, Toglia JU (1981) Medial frontal cortex infarction and the alien hand sign. Arch Neurol 38:683–686

Hécaen H, Albert ML (1978) Human neuropsychology. New York, John Wiley & Sons

Ingvar DH (1985) "Memory of the future:" An essay on the temporal organization of conscious awareness. Human Neurobiol 4:127–136

Jackson JH (1915) On affections of speech from disease of the brain. Brain 38:107–174

Jacobsen CF (1935) Functions of the frontal association area in primates. Arch Neurol Psychiatry 33:558–569

Jonides J, Smith EE, Doeppe RA, Awh E, Minoshima S, Mintun MA (1993) Spatial working memory in humans as revealed by PET. Nature 363:623–625

Kornhuber HH, Deecke L (1965) Hirnpotentialänderungen bei Willkürbewegungen und passiven Bewegungen des Menschen: Bereitschaftspotential und reafferent Potentiale. Pfluegers Arch Gesamte Physiol 284:1–17

Lashley KS (1951) The problem of serial order in behavior. In: Jeffress LA (ed) Cerebral mechanisms in behavior. New York, John Wiley & Sons, pp 112–146

Lewinsohn PM, Zieler RE, Libet J, Eyeberg S, Nielson G (1972) Short-term memory: A comparison between frontal and nonfrontal right- and left-hemisphere brain damaged patients. J Comp Physiol Psychol 81:248–255

Lhermitte F, Deroulsne J, Signoret JL (1972) Analyse neuropsychologique du syndrome frontal. Rev Neurol 127:415–440

Libet B (1985) Unconscious cerebral initiative and the role of conscious will in voluntary action. Behav Brain Sci 8:529–566

Luria AR (1966) Higher cortical functions in man. New York, Basic Books

Luria AR (1970) Traumatic aphasia. The Hague, Mouton

Milner B, Petrides M, Smith ML (1985) Frontal lobes and the temporal organization of memory. Human Neurobiol 4:137–142

Niki H (1974) Differential activity of prefrontal units during right and left delayed response trials. Brain Res 70:346–349

Pandya DN, Yeterian EH (1985) Architecture and connections of cortical association areas. In: Peters A, Jones EG (eds) Association and auditory cortices. New York, Plenum, pp 3–61

Quintana J, Fuster JM (1992) Mnemonic and predictive functions of cortical neurons in a memory task. NeuroReport 3:721–724

Shindy WW, Posley KA, Fuster JM (1994) Reversibel deficit in haptic delay tasks from cooling prefrontal cortex. Cerebral Cortex 4:443–450

Sierra-Paredes G, Fuster JM (1993) Auditory-visual association task impaired by cooling prefrontal cortex. Soc Neurosci Abstracts 19:801 (Abstract)

Stuss DT, Benson DF (1986) The frontal lobes. New York, Raven Press

Swartz BE, Halgren E, Fuster JM, Simplins F, Gee M, Mandelkern M (1995) Cortical metabolic activation in humans during a visual memory task. Cerebral Cortex, in press

Tanji J, Evarts EV (1976) Anticipatory activity of motor cortex neurons in relation to direction of an intended movement. J Neurophysiol 39:1060–1068

Thompson RF (1986) The neurobiology of learning and memory. Science 233:941–947

Walter WG, Cooper R, Aldrige VJ, McCallum WC, Winter AL (1964) Contingent negative variation: An electric sign of sensori-motor association and expectancy in the the human brain. Nature 203:380–384

Weizsäcker VVon (1950) Der Gestaltkreis. Stuttgart, Thieme

Neural Mechanisms Supporting Successful Social Decisions in Simians

M. Raleigh[1,2,3,4], M. McGuire[1,2,3], W. Melega[3,4,5], S. Cherry[5,6], S.-C. Huang[4,5,6], and M. Phelps[3,4,5,6]

Summary

Vervet monkeys are an appropriate species to model aspects of the neurobiology of human social decision-making. Vervets are phylogenetically closely related to human beings and possess large brains that show substantial postnatal maturation, exhibit rich behavioral repertoires, and establish enduring and complex social relationships. This chapter describes two types of investigations that examined the links between monoaminergic neurotransmitter systems, frontal lobe function, and effective social decision-making in vervet monkeys. One set examined indices of serotonergic function while the other utilized positron emission tomography (PET) to evaluate cerebral glucose metabolism.

Serotonergic systems have been implicated in mediating the social behavior decisions necessary to acquire high social status among adult animals. In vervet monkeys, under appropriate social conditions, pharmacologically enhancing serotonergic function dramatically facilitated the likelihood of becoming dominant. Adult male monkeys treated with fluoxetine or tryptophan exhibited enhanced abilities to evaluate and act more effectively than their vehicle-treated rivals. Treated subjects engaged in more effective aggression, formed and maintained more reciprocal alliances, and were more likely to initiate sequences of behavior that led to both attacks against and the ostracism of rival group members. Pharmacologically diminished serotonergic function induced behavioral changes in the opposite direction. In addition, neuroanatomical studies suggest that lifelong, individual differences in initiating appropriate, effective aggression, engaging in prosocial behavior, and participating in joint cooperative actions correlate strongly with the density (B_{max}) of serotonin-2A (S_{2A}) receptors in the posterior orbitofrontal cortex, the amygdala, and the temporal pole.

[1] Department of Psychiatry, UCLA School of Medicine, Los Angeles, CA 90024, USA
[2] Brain Research Institute, UCLA School of Medicine, Los Angeles, CA 90024, USA
[3] Nonhuman Primate Research Laboratory, Research Service, Sepulveda Veterans Administration Medical Center Sepulveda, CA 91343, USA
[4] Department of Energy, Laboratory of Structural Biology, UCLA, Los Angeles, CA 90024, USA
[5] Department of Molecular and Medical Pharmacology, UCLA School of Medicine, Los Angeles, CA 90024, USA
[6] Crump Institute for Biological Imaging, UCLA School of Medicine, Los Angeles, CA 90024, USA

A.R. Damasio et al. (Eds.)
Neurobiology of Decision-Making
© Springer-Verlag Berlin Heidelberg 1996

A second set of studies used positron emission tomography (PET) to examine the acute and enduring effects of early cognitive enrichment on brain metabolism and behavior. While in their social group, young animals were systematically exposed to cognitive tasks for 30 consecutive days. Relative to age- and sex-matched controls who were not exposed to cognitive enrichment, these subjects showed increased rates of glucose metabolism in selected neocortical regions, notably the dorsolateral and orbital frontal cortex. Other regions, such as the brain stem and cerebellum, did not show similar increases in glucose metabolism. This regionally specific, increased metabolic rate persisted for 15 months following the termination of cognitive enrichment. Further, enriched subjects continued to out-perform control subjects not only on cognitive tasks but also on social problems. They were less distressed by novelty, more effective at evaluating challenging social situations, and more likely to make the types of social decisions that enable individuals to attain high social status. These observations suggest that there may be substantial plasticity in the neural systems essential to making effective social decisions.

These two sets of investigations support and extend observations made on normal and neurologically impaired human beings. They suggest that serotonergic systems, particularly those terminating in the frontal cortex, may underlie stable individual differences in the ability to make effective social decisions. They also imply that early cognitive enrichment may affect social decision-making processes in addition to having enduring effects on neural function.

Introduction

Much of our research has focused on the neural mechanisms that support effective social decision-making in nonhuman primates. As adults, socially living monkeys exhibit substantial individual differences in their capacities to attain high rank, to form and maintain affiliative bonds, and to integrate effectively into new social settings. In both vervet monkeys and rhesus macaques many of these individual differences may be due to individual differences in monoaminergic neurotrans-mitter systems (Botchin et al. 1993; Higley et al. 1993; Kaplan et al. 1995; Raleigh and McGuire 1994). Behavioral observations suggest that serotonergic systems may be particularly important in the mediation of stable individual behavioral differences. Further, pharmacological studies that experimentally manipulate monoaminergic function suggest that serotonergic systems enhance the ability to make the behavioral decisions necessary to attain high social rank (Raleigh et al. 1991).

Lesion studies in monkeys and clinical observations in human beings indicate that specific brain regions are involved in the mediation of social behavior (Adolph et al., this volume; Damasio 1994; Damasio et al. 1994; Fuster 1989; Pandya and Yeterian, this volume). These regions include the amygdala, portions of the frontal cortex, and the temporal pole. There are intriguing links in monkeys between the density of serotonin 2A (S_{2A}) receptors in these regions and persistent, lifelong patterns of social behavior. Individuals that have a high density of S_{2A} receptors in these regions exhibit substantially less destructive, aggressive behavior over the course of their lifetime. These individuals are also particularly adept at engaging other animals in positive, prosocial behavioral interactions. Further, the density of S_{2A} receptors in the orbitofrontal cortex correlates positively with the ability to participate in cooperative behavior. Thus, in adults, lesion and anatomical studies suggest that a particular transmitter system, serotonin, operating in a particular brain region, the orbitofrontal cortex, may underlie lifelong individual differences in the ability to make effective social decisions.

Although there are persistent individual differences in behavior among adult monkeys and human beings, there also appears to be substantial plasticity in the neural systems that contribute to effective social decision-making. In rodents (Greenough 1992) and human beings (Jacobs and Scheibel 1993), neocortical areas are particularly sensitive to environmental enrichment. Based on these and other studies (Bryan and Riessen 1989; Bourgeois et al. 1994; Clarke et al. 1994; Freidman and Goldman-Rakic 1994; Goldman-Rakic 1993; Martin et al. 1991; Rakic et al. 1986), we have begun to investigate whether enriched, structured learning results in persistent increases in brain glucose metabolism and in enduring alterations in behavior. Preliminary evidence suggests that this type of enrichment does indeed lead to regionally specific increases in brain glucose metabolism and in fact is also accompanied by long-term alterations in behavior. Such enriched animals are more likely to attain high status, accommodate expeditiously to novelty, and engage in cooperative behavior.

Thus at present there is evidence for both stability in the neural systems that underlie effective social decision-making among adults and plasticity in these systems among developing animals. The current chapter highlights some of these findings in monkeys. After enumerating some of the features of vervet monkeys that make them well suited for these studies, we will describe the links between serotonin and effective social decision-making. Subsequently, we comment on the enduring metabolic and behavioral effects of structured enrichment during early experience. We conclude by speculating on how monkey studies may inform studies of the neurobiology of social decision-making in human beings.

Nonhuman Primate Models

Our studies have used vervet monkeys to evaluate the links among monoaminergic neurotransmitter systems, neuroplasticity, and social decision-making. These studies take advantage of our large primate research colony that currently houses more than 550 vervet monkeys living in 22 social groups. Animals in this colony have known pedigrees and exhibit a wide range of individual differences in social behavior, endocrine profiles, and indirect indices of brain monoamine function (obtained by measuring the concentration of monoamine metabolites in cerebrospinal fluid). Since this colony was established, normative behavioral and physiological data have been obtained from a large number of developing, mature, and aged monkeys (Fairbanks and McGuire 1988; Raleigh and McGuire 1994). These normative data provide baseline information which permits a more completely detailed evaluation of the acute and enduring effects of pharmacological and behavioral interventions.

Ethical and practical considerations constrain comprehensive, prospective studies of the effects of gender, age, and epigenetic influences on functional brain maturation in humans. Consequently, it is crucial to develop animal models in which the contributions of particular neurotransmitters to social decision-making can be examined experimentally. Nonhuman primates exhibit rich repertoires of social and individual behavior that parallel many aspects of human non-verbal behavior. They are the among the most appropriate subjects for research into the postnatal "mechanisms underlying human sensory and motor capacities, perception, learning, memory, reasoning, cognition, and cerebral dominance" (King et al. 1988, p. 1476). The development of visual, motor, and social skills has been examined in baboons, macaques, vervets, and other species (Castell and Sackett 1973; Fragazy and Adams-Curtis 1991; Gunderson et al. 1993; Harlow 1969; Higley et al. 1992a; Mason et al. 1993; Rosenblum and Paully 1984; Struhsaker 1971; Westergaard 1993). Comparative investigations have identified the parallels in the development of basic perceptual, motor, and cognitive abilities in monkey and human infants. Parallel development has been observed in a wide range of areas including visual responsiveness, cross-modal recognition, and object concept (Andrews and Rosenblum 1993; Gibson 1991; Jacobs and Scheibel 1993; Suomi 1991). Gunderson and Sackett (1984) suggested that there was a consistent ratio in the developmental rates of monkeys and humans: one month of postnatal maturation in the monkey was equivalent to approximately four months in humans. This ontogenetic relationship is important for establishing comparative norms in primate models of human neural development.

As shown in Table 1, our observations on vervet monkeys have delineated a set of behavioral milestones that the animals attain in a particular order within fairly discrete time frames. Although the timing of some events may vary between

Table 1. Major behavioral and motor milestones in developing vervet monkeys

Age (months)	Behavioral characteristics
0–2	Grasp, startle, nutritive sucking reflexes present. Completely dependent on mother. Sleep is predominant activity. Continual contact with mother.
3–6	Breaks maternal contact. Sleep declines. Eats solid food. Social play and exploration begin. Visually recognizes individuals.
7–12	Less maternal dependence. Climbing, swinging, running develop fully. Sex differences in play apparent.
13–24	Younger sibling born. Sex differences in affiliative and aggressive behavior appear. Females begin to form alliances that will persist through life.
25–36	Onset of puberty with associated behavioral and endocrine changes.
37–48	Young adulthood.

individuals, the sequential order appears to be invariant across subjects and species typical (see also Kraemer 1992; Ruppenthal and Sackett 1992; Schneider 1992). These sequential changes are characterized by declining physical dependence on the mother and increasing visual, motor, and social independence. These behavioral landmarks parallel what has been reported in other species and in free-ranging conditions (Cheney and Seyfarth 1983; Fairbanks and McGuire 1988; Higley et al. 1992b; Isbell 1990; Simpson and Howe 1988).

In contrast to humans, the monkeys' diet, alcohol consumption, drug use, and other environmental factors that might substantially affect development and brain metabolism can be controlled experimentally. Lifelong patterns of social, motor, and cognitive behavior can be directly monitored rather than being reconstructed through interviews or other indirect procedures (Amaral 1993; Brown and Linnoila 1990; Higley et al. 1992b; Kraemer et al. 1989). Many of the cognitive, perceptual, and sensorimotor changes that characterize the infant monkey's emerging behavioral capacities have been associated with ontogenetic anatomical and metabolic changes in the monkey brain (Bourgeois et al. 1985; Clark et al. 1988; Diamond and Goldman-Rakic 1989; Goldman-Rakic 1988; Goldman-Rakic and Brown 1982; Kennedy et al. 1982; O'Kusky and Colonnier 1982; Rakic et al. 1986). In our studies, we are particularly interested in extending these findings by focusing on the development of complex social skills (Cheney et al. 1986; Cheney and Seyfarth 1990) and specific changes in brain metabolism.

Relative to other non-human primates, vervet monkeys offer several research advantages. First, they are abundant and tolerate captivity well. The large number of animals available makes it possible to use histochemical and biochemical analyses to directly test inferences drawn from non-invasive imaging and physiological studies. Second, compared to many other Old World monkeys, vervets exhibit relatively little sexual dimorphism in terms of body size. As adults, females are approximately 80% of the body weight and 85% of the length of males. These measurements resemble the magnitude of sexual dimorphism observed in humans and are less than those found in baboons, gorillas, and macaques.

Third, vervets manifest sex differences in behavior that parallel those seen in human beings. Among vervet monkeys these differences, particularly in play patterns emerge during the second half of the first year of life. Juvenile male vervets spend more time engaged in rough and tumble play than do females and, when given the opportunity, young males prefer male peers as play partners. By contrast, females distribute their play among age peers of both sexes and among younger juveniles. The sex differences in the rate and form of play support the hypotheses that, among males, play functions to hone fighting skills. Adult male vervet monkeys are more dependent on individual fighting skills than are adult females. Juvenile female vervets also frequently engage in activities that may enhance their likelihood of being reproductively successful as adults. Such activities include play mothering and establishing long-term relationships with adult females (Berman 1992; Cheney and Seyfarth 1983; Fairbanks 1993; Raleigh and McGuire 1990). Prior to puberty sex differences in behavior are present, but at puberty they become pronounced. In vervets and other Old World monkeys, puberty is characterized by dramatic behavioral, anatomical, and physiological changes (Bernstein et al. 1991;

Pfaff 1982; Plant 1988). In free ranging settings, vervet males between 3 and 5 years of age migrate out of their natal groups and attempt to join other social groups. This transfer process presents a difficult challenge during which animals encounter novel stimuli, forge new social relationships, rely on their individual fighting skills, face increased risk of predation, and solve demanding cognitive problems. Between 30% and 60% of the males do not migrate successfully and probably die, perhaps from predation or disease (Cheney and Seyfarth 1983; Isbell 1990). In contrast to males, female vervet monkeys typically remain in their natal groups. Among females, the attainment of high rank and reproductive success also seems to depend on cognitive abilities and social competence. As they mature, females become increasingly reliant on their ability to form social alliances and to correctly anticipate and respond to social challenges.

A fourth feature is that vervets mature about a year sooner than do macaques. Females can reproduce at 2.5 years. Males reach full stature with completely developed secondary sexual characteristics by age five. These compressed developmental periods shorten the time needed to conduct lifelong prospective studies.

Fifth, vervet monkeys are being used in a growing number of neurobehavioral studies and some of these investigations suggest that vervets and human beings exhibit similar sex differences in the concentration of cerebrospinal fluid monoamine metabolites. In humans, the concentrations of CSF 5-HIAA and HVA are indirect indices of global brain serotonergic and dopaminergic turnover. Most human studies suggest that the concentration of these metabolites are higher in women than in men. Similar sex differences are seen in vervet monkeys but have not been uniformly found in macaques (Argen et al. 1986; Brown and Linnoila 1990; Higley et al. 1993; Raleigh et al. 1992; Shelton et al. 1988). Vervets and humans also show similar regional differences in the concentrations of subtypes of serotonergic receptors. For example in both species, there is a rostral/caudal and cortex/subcortical gradient in S_{2A} receptors (Brammer et al. 1987; Charney et al. 1990). More generally, the distribution of monoamines in vervet and rhesus monkeys more closely resembles that seen in human beings, and all three primate species exhibit important contrasts with rodents. (Peroutka 1988; Sanders-Bush 1988; Williams and Goldman-Rakic 1993; Wilson and Molliver 1991).

Serotonergic Mechanisms

In monkeys, apes, and human beings, rank has both its privileges and its obligations. Relative to subordinate animals, high-ranking animals have preferential access to limited resources such as food, preferred sleeping sites, shelter, and desired social partners. In addition to rank-related behavioral differences, dominant and subordinate adults also appear to differ physiologically. For example, among subordinate adult female marmosets, ovulation is suppressed, probably because of the absence of an LH surge (Abbott 1987). In free-ranging baboon groups, high- and low-ranking adult males differ in the hormonal output from their hypothalamic-adrenal cortical axis. High-ranking male baboons show lower basal cortisol, yet exhibit large cortisol responses to the challenges of capture, to dexamethasone, and to cortisol-releasing factor (Sapolsky 1990). Dominant and subordinate vervet monkeys may also differ in their social decision-making. For example, when confronted by a threat from a juvenile group member, dominant individuals are more likely than subordinate animals to look at the juvenile's mother, approach and sit near the mother, or attempt to engage the infant in affiliative behavior. By contrast, subordinate vervets are more likely to threaten or ignore the juvenile. Dominant male vervets may also be more flexible in solving other social problems, including the ability to enlist allies in aggressive encounters. However, the relationship between rank and cognitive performance is less clear. Although dominant animals may exceed subordinate animals on maze and other cognitive tasks, it is unclear if these differences are secondary to status-linked differences in anxiety, mood, or some other factor.

In stable social settings, correlative studies suggest that some of the rank-related differences in social decision-making may be due to differences in serotonergic function. Experimental treatment with drugs that enhance serotonergic function support this view. Such treatments lead to increases in affiliative behavior, increases in the likelihood of using multiple strategies to re-spond to provocative challenges from intruders, and increases in performance on selected cognitive tasks. However, in stable social groups, traditional relationships and expectations may constrain or limit a subject's behavioral and cognitive op-tions. In view of the conservative nature of social relationships in stable monkey groups, it is not surprising that drug-induced increases in serotonergic function do not result in subordinate animals becoming dominant. However, when dominance relationships become unstable (as, for example, following the removal of the high-est ranking male from the group), individual differences in the capacity to activate serotonergic systems is one of the key factors in determining which animal will become dominant.

In a series of studies, we examined the effects of pharmacological manipula-tion of serotonergic function in social groups from which the dominant males had been removed (Raleigh et al. 1991). In a cross-over, vehicle-controlled study, dominant males were removed from their social group. During the next four weeks, one of the remaining subordinate males received drugs intended to pro-mote or diminish brain serotonergic function. The serotonin precursor tryptophan and the serotonin reuptake inhibitor, fluoxetine, were used to augment serotonergic function (Fuller 1992; Young and Teff 1989). Serotonergic function was diminished chronically by the use of the serotonin antagonists fenfluramine and cyproheptadine. Administered acutely, fenfluramine releases serotonin from presynatic vesicles and may act as an indirect agonist. However, administered chronically, fenfluramine disrupts serotonergic storage vesicles, diminishes tryptophan hydroxylase activity, decreases CSF 5-HIAA and brain serotonin con-centrations and produces behavioral effects compatible with decrease serotonergic function (Appel et al. 1990; Fuller 1992; Peroutka 1988; Sanders-Bush 1988; Wagner and Peroutka 1990).

When the 12 treated males received tryptophan or fluoxetine, they became dominant; when they received drugs that diminished serotonergic function, they did not become dominant. The sequence and timing of the behavioral changes paralleled those seen in naturalistic conditions (Raleigh et al. 1991). Thus, there was an initial increase in affiliative interactions with females, followed by increase in female support in coalitions against the remaining male group members, and finally the systematic defeat of the remaining males in dyadic aggressive encounters. As shown in Table 2, the treated males also showed changes in behaviors that were indicative of an enhanced capacity to make effective social decisions: their latency to respond to positive social overtures decreased; they were more likely to approach and sit near distressed group members; and they were less likely to attack others without first soliciting help from other group members. Fenfluramine and cyproheptadine treatment produced behavioral effects in the opposite direction to those of fluoxetine and tryptophan. When receiving fenfluramine and cyproheptadine, subjects showed decreases in affiliative behavior, increases in aggression, and decrements in the likelihood of responding to positive social overtures. Treatment with drugs that enhanced noradrenergic function failed to produce analogous effects on dominance acquisition. These observations strongly suggest that when hierarchical relationships are uncertain, the activation of serotonergic mechanisms may be a critical first step in the expression of the behavioral actions and decision-making capabilities that permit an individual to attain high dominance status.

Based on this and other observations, we thought that many of the stable individual differences in temperament and overt behavioral styles that persist from adolescence to adulthood may be linked to individual differences in the density of S_{2A} receptors. We tested this hypothesis by determining the affinity (K_m) and density (B_{max}) of S_{2A} receptors in 13 different cortical and subcortical areas. As shown in Table 3, S_{2A} receptor density in the posterior orbitofrontal, medial frontal, and amygdala was inversely related to the likelihood of engaging in destructive

Table 2. Serotonin and effective social behavior[1]

Behavioral pattern	Enhanced	Vehicle	Diminished
Respond to overtures	12.5 ± 1.7*	8.3 ± 1.1	5.3 ± 1.2*
Approach distressed group members	16.2 ± 1.9*	7.2 ± 1.1	6.9 ± 1.0
Attack without soliciting	16.1 ± 11.1*	37.2 ± 1.1	36.9 ± 1.0

[1] The effects of enhancing or diminishing serotonergic function on three behavioral measures that are indicative of the ability to engage in effective social behavior. Serotonergic activity was increased by the administration of either fluoxetine (2 mg/kg/day) or tryptophan (40 mg/kg/day) and diminished by fenfluramine (2 mg/kg/day) or cyproheptadine (60 ug/kg/day), as described elsewhere (Raleigh et al. 1991). The table presents the rates (events/hr) at which the subjects responded to positive social overtures from others and approached distressed group members. The data on attacking others are the percentage of total aggressive encounters initiated by the subjects that occurred without first soliciting support from other group members. An asterisk (*) indicates that the rate of behavior during treatment differs from the rate under vehicle conditions by Scheffe's test (p < 0.05).

Table 3. Individual differences in S_{2A} receptors and behavior[1]

Area	Mean (SD)	Min	Max	Aggress	Prosocial	Cooperation
Orbitofrontal Cortex	145 (25)	98	200	0.27	0.26	0.31
Posterior Orbitofrontal Cortex	132 (42)	67	193	−0.74*	0.86*	0.65*
Superior Frontal Cortex	127 (41)	27	194	0.19	0.19	−0.21
Medial Frontal Cortex	128 (31)	81	185	−0.63*	0.14	−0.23
Inferior Frontal Cortex	116 (31)	70	173	0.32	−0.22	−0.18
Parietal Cortex	105 (15)	84	135	0.30	0.35	−0.28
Occipital Cortex	95 (33)	25	137	0.25	−0.09	0.09
Temporal Pole	114 (39)	38	179	−0.41	0.70*	0.64*
Amygdala	54 (32)	10	118	−0.61*	0.63*	0.30
Hippocampus	45 (18)	12	77	−0.34	0.63*	−0.23
Midbrain	13 (7)	0	22	0.13	−0.22	0.07
Hypothalamus	34 (13)	18	65	0.22	−0.25	−0.21
Thalamus	19 (10)	0	40	0.19	0.40	0.29
Raphe	7 (6)	0	15	0.07	0.15	0.13

[1] Individual differences in S_{2A} receptor density (B_{max}) and lifelong differences in behavior. Data are from 16 adult male vervet monkeys. S_{2A} receptor density was determined by measuring ketanserin binding (see Brammer et al. 1986). Brain areas are described in detail elsewhere (Brammer et al. 1986). The Mean (SD), Min, and Max refer to the mean (and standard deviation), the minimal and maximal values among the 16 subjects. Units are femtomoles/mg protein. Aggress, Prosocial, and Cooperation refer to initiating injurious aggression, engaging in positive social behavior, and participating in cooperative social actions. Numbers in these columns represent the Pearson product moment correlation between the density of S_{2A} receptor and the behavior. An asterisk (*) indicates $p < 0.05$.

aggressive behavior. The density of S_{2A} binding sites in the posterior orbitofrontal, hippocampus, amygdala, and temporal pole also correlated with engaging in positive, prosocial behavior. Cooperation involved participating with another group member to attain a food reward or to joining with a group member in aggressing against a potentially intruding extra-group member. Engaging in cooperative behavior correlated with the density of S_{2A} receptors in the posterior orbitofrontal and temporal pole. These observations suggest that there are regional differences in the contributions of serotonergic systems to the inhibition of aggression, to the expression of prosocial behavior, and to the promotion of the participation in cooperative behavior. These data implicate the posterior orbitofrontal cortex as one area particularly involved in the expression of effective social decision-making.

Neuroplasticity

Many of our previous studies have focused on lifelong, persistent individual differences in the behavioral styles exhibited by adult monkeys. Such differences may represent nonhuman primate analogs to the concepts of temperament and personality (Cloninger 1987; McGuire et al. 1994; Virkkunen et al. 1994). However, in addition to persistent individual differences in temperament, we are also interested in plasticity. We have begun to examine whether structured, visual-motor learning during early development induces short-term and enduring alterations in brain glucose metabolism and whether these enriched animals exhibit persistent behavioral changes indicative of enhanced social decision-making.

These investigations build on and extend prior examinations of primate neurobehavioral development, behavioral ontogeny, and neuroplasticity. For example, the time course of histological changes in the developing monkey brain has been documented in considerable detail. Neocortical synaptic and neurotransmitter receptor densities increase sharply during the last two months of the six-month-long gestation, peaking between two and four months postnatally, and then declining gradually to adult values (Bourgeois 1993; Bourgeois et al. 1989; Lidow et al. 1991; Lidow and Rakic 1992; Meinecke and Rakic 1992; Rakic et al. 1986; Shaw et al. 1991; Wenk et al. 1989; Zecevic et al. 1989; Zecevic and Rakic 1991). In the monkey neocortex, synaptic density peaks at 30–50% above adult values. This peak may occur synchronously in different neocortical regions.

Histological data indicate that the period around the fourth month of post-natal life in Old World monkeys is characterized by a plateau in synaptic and monoamine receptor density in neocortex, followed by a selective elimination of synapses. Synaptogenesis in the molecular layer of the rhesus dentate gyrus also attains a peak in the fourth and fifth postnatal months, a time that corresponds to the increase in asymmetrical synapses and dendritic spine density. Synaptic density in this area then decreases to adult values by 10 months (Duffy and Rakic 1983; Eckenhoff and Rakic 1991). In the neostriatum, synaptic density reaches a plateau at the beginning of the second postnatal month and is maintained at this level through adulthood (Brand and Rakic 1984). Qualitative and quantitative analyses have shown that dendritic systems in the visual cortex of *Macaca nemestria* monkeys exhibit marked increases in spine density within the first two months of postnatal life (Boothe et al. 1985).

The period of excess synaptic density in specific neural areas may correlate with the emergence of the principal functions mediated by these areas. For example, in comparing local cerebral metabolic rate for glucose (LCMRGlc) between newborn and adult rhesus monkeys, Kennedy et al. (1982) found a relationship between LCMRGlc increases in a particular brain structure and the emergence of behavior at least in part mediated by that structure. LCMRGlc rates in neonatal monkeys were lower than pubescent rates in structures superior to the midbrain, particularly striate and inferior temporal cortex. In contrast, LCMRGlc rates in neonatal auditory and somatosensory cortical areas were similar to pubescent rates. This pattern of glucose utilization correlated with the behavioral capabilities of neonatal monkeys, whose auditory and tactile abilities are more advanced than their visual abilities.

Similar relationships between LCMRGlc or local cerebral blood flow (LCBF) ontogeny and behavioral maturation have also been observed in dogs (Duffy et al. 1979; Gregoire et al. 1981), sheep (Abrams et al. 1984), rats (Nehlig et al. 1988), and cats (Chugani et al. 1991). In general, phylogenetically older structures (e.g., brainstem, cerebellum, thalamus) seem to demonstrate considerable metabolic maturity compared to telencephalic structures in the neonatal period. Hence, the newborn's behavior may be dominated by these structures and is therefore relatively unsophisticated. As the animal matures, phylogenetically newer regions in the brain become more functionally active, and the animal achieves greater behavioral complexity. Based on these metabolic-behavioral relationships, Kennedy et al. (1982) hypothesized that a developmental rise in the resting metabolic rate of a particular neuroanatomical structure signals the time when that structure contributes to the behavioral repertoire of the species.

Attractive as this structural-function hypothesis was, there was no suitable method to test it longitudinally in humans or other primates until the development of positron emission tomography (PET). PET is a noninvasive imaging modality that can be used to measure local chemical functions in various body organs (Phelps et al. 1986) by employing tracer kinetic measurements of compounds labeled with positron-emitting isotopes. The technique allows the direct measurement of regional glucose utilization (Mori et al. 1990; Sokoloff et al. 1977, 1994) and thus can provide a noninvasive means of documenting the acute and enduring effects of enrichment.

Obtaining longitudinal LCMRGlc data as the monkeys pass through behaviorally defined stages will aid in linking alterations in brain metabolism to the emergence of behavioral and cognitive milestones. The availability of such normative data may facilitate the assessment of the metabolic effects of enrichment. Based on preliminary PET studies, it is possible to trace the ontogenetic course of LCMRGlc in particular structures. For instance, Figure 1 shows the developmental course of LCMRGlc in the dorsolateral frontal cortex, an area which is of particular interest because of its contributions to cognitive and social skills (Goldman-Rakic 1988). LCMRGlc is lowest in animals less than three months of age, peaks between the third and sixth months and then declines to adulthood. At the onset of adolescence (months 29–31) LCMRGlc appears to show another transient peak. Four-year-old animals did not differ from fully adult monkeys (8 to 11 years). These observations are compatible with the view that exposing subjects to enrichment regimes when subjects are four to eight months of age may be particularly effective in inducing persistent, long-term metabolic changes.

Pilot data suggest that particular types of visual motor experience in young monkeys may result in regionally specific increases in LCMRGlc. In preliminary studies, three six-month-old monkeys were exposed to complex foraging and structured visual motor learning tasks for 1 hr/day for 31 days. Subjects actively tended to and manipulated these stimuli. Age-matched control subjects could see and touch but not manipulate or solve the puzzles.

PET scans were obtained prior to (at 5.5 months) and after (at 8.5 months) exposure to the visual motor stimulation in some of the experimental and the control subjects. During 2-deoxy-2 [18F] fluoro-D-glucose (FDG) uptake, subjects were awake and fully conscious, thereby obviating concerns arising from anesthesia. Figure 2 shows that the pattern of glucose metabolism differs between enriched and control subjects.

Table 4 shows that enrichment during a critical period of development is

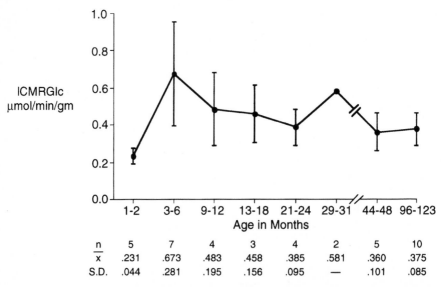

n	5	7	4	3	4	2	5	10
x̄	.231	.673	.483	.458	.385	.581	.360	.375
S.D.	.044	.281	.195	.156	.095	—	.101	.085

Fig. 1. Ontogenetic changes in LCMRGlc in the dorsolateral prefrontal cortex, an area that appears to be particularly important in the mediation of cognitive and social skills (Goldman-Rakic 1988; Fuster 1989). LCMRGlc is lowest in animals less than three months of age, peaks between the third and sixth months, and then declines to adulthood. Seemingly at the onset of adolescence (months 29–31) LCMRGlc shows another transient peak. Four-year-old animals did not differ from fully adult monkeys (8 to 11 years)

associated with regionally specific increments in LCMRGlc. One month after exposure to the task had ended, the experimental subjects showed increases in the dorsolateral frontal, and orbitofrontal cortices of 35% and 28% respectively. Other regions, including the thalamus and the brain stem, were unchanged. In contrast to the experimental subjects, the control animals manifested slight decrements in the three cortical areas.

This observation suggests that specific visual motor experience, including engaging in cognitive tasks, may indeed induce enduring regionally specific increases in LCMRGlc. Phylogenetically more recently evolved systems appear to be more sensitive to stimulation than older regions. PET data also suggest that there may also be enduring metabolic consequences of this enrichment. One set of these animals have been followed for 24 months after enrichment and they continue to show enhanced, regionally specific increases in brain metabolism over a period of time corresponding to about nine years of human life.

There also appear to be enduring behavioral effects of this enrichment. After enrichment has ceased, enriched subjects outperform control animals on a battery of cognitive tests. Further, the effects of this cognitive enrichment appear to extend into the realm of social behavior as well. Thus, relative to the normal developmental patterns obtained from 130 animals, enriched subjects rank in the top 5% for engaging in reciprocal play, establishing alliances, and using aggression effectively. Developmental studies suggest that these are the harbingers of achieving

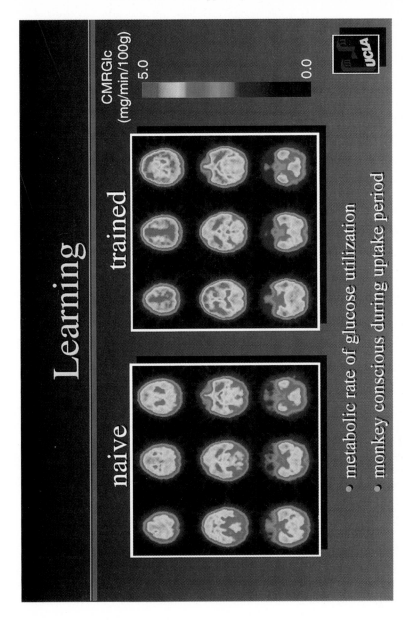

Fig. 2. Effects of enrichment on LCMRGlc. LCMRGlc in horizontal planes in an enriched and a control subject. The figure illustrates the increased rates of LCMRGLc in the experimental subject's frontal and other cortical areas

Table 4. Effects of visual motor enrichment on LCMRGlc. PET scans were obtained prior to and after exposure to the visual motor stimulation in three experimental and six control subjects. During FDG uptake, subjects were awake and fully conscious. Data are from five regions of interest and show that this experience during a critical period of development is associated with regionally specific increments in LCMRGlc. One month after exposure to the task had ended, experimental subjects showed increases in the dorsolateral frontal, and orbitofrontal of 35% and 28%, respectively. Other regions, including the thalamus and the brain stem, were unchanged

Region	Subject	LCMRGIc (umol/min/gm)		
		Pre	Post	Change
Dorsolateral frontal	Exp	0.659	0.892	35%
	Control	0.713	0.681	−3%
Orbitofrontal	Exp	0.630	0.806	28%
	Control	0.660	0.641	3%
Primary visual	Exp	0.637	0.668	5%
	Control	0.601	0.570	−5%
Thalamus	Exp	0.429	0.449	5%
	Control	0.493	0.502	2%
Brain stem	Exp	0.469	0.478	2%
	Control	0.494	0.508	3%

high scores on rating systems that assess social competence among adults (McGuire et al. 1994). Subjects undergoing enrichment as infants are likely to exhibit enhanced social competence as adults and these behavioral effects may be the result of metabolic changes in frontal and other regions.

Conclusions

These and other studies of the neural systems supporting social decision-making in monkeys (Brothers and Ring 1993) may inform investigations of human beings in at least three ways. First, they suggest that individual differences among normal human beings in social decision-making may be supported by individual differences in serotonergic systems. Most examinations of the links between monoamines and behavior among human beings test for differences between diagnostic groups. For example, studies of patients with obsessive compulsive disorders (Insel and Winslow 1992) suggest there are differences in serotonergic function between this group of patients and control populations. As a group, patients with manic depressive disease may exhibit alterations in noradrenergic activity. Although the focus of human studies has largely been on differences between diagnostic groups, there are nonetheless substantial individual differences among members of diagnostic groups and within the normal population. Such individual differences have rarely been the focus of systematic investigation. With the development of functional imaging procedures and the refinement of rating scales that can measure social competence, it may become possible to identify the contributions of serotonin and other monoamines to social effectiveness in normal as well as neurologically impaired individuals.

Second, monkey studies suggest that more attention should be directed to the neural systems that support gender-based differences in brain metabolism. Given the scope of the behavioral sex differences in monkeys, apes, and human beings, it is likely that there are corresponding sex-linked differences in brain metabolism. The recognition and documentation of both differences and similarities between females and males is critical in order to avoid overly simplistic generalizations about the links between regional differences in brain metabolism and social decision-making. The metabolic processes occurring in the brains of male monkeys and male human beings may not serve as particularly incisive models of female brain metabolism.

Third, it is becoming increasingly apparent that normative, baseline data are critical in order to more fully assess acute and long-term effects of specific interventions on the neural systems supporting social decision-making. Documenting the normal developmental course of neural ontogeny is critical for the interpretation of the short- and long-term effects of experimental interventions on neuroplasticity, reorganization, and compensation in both normal and brain-damaged children. For example, descriptive and correlative data from PET studies of children indicate that the LCMRGlc rates of most cortical brain regions at birth are about 70% of adult rates. These rates rise rapidly to reach adult levels by 2 years and are about twice adult values by 3–4 years. High rates are maintained until about 10 years when they gradually decline to adult levels by the end of the second decade (Chugani and Phelps 1986; Chugani et al. 1987; Chugani et al. 1991). The observation that children, in contrast to adults, can sustain damage to large areas of the brain but show remarkably little functional deficit is generally attributed to the reorganization capability of the developing brain. Between 8 and 10 years, when LCMRGlc rates for many cortical regions begins to decline, there is a notable decrease in both the recovery and sparing of function following injury to the child's brain. The relationship between maturational trends, neuroplasticity, and social decision-making seen in monkeys suggests that the maximal effect of interventions in human beings may correspond to the time in development when LCMRGlc rates and other indices of neuroplasticity are maximal.

Acknowledgments. The research reported in this chapter has benefited from the outstanding technical support of Deborah B. Pollack, Grenvill Morton, Maureen Sinclair, Wendye Marcowitz, Vishad Nibali, Judy Edwards, David Youssefzadeh, David Stout, Dan Dekeman, and Valde Ladno. The research was supported by the Research Service of the Veterans Administration Medical Center, Sepulveda; the Harry Frank Guggenheim Foundation, the Department of Energy Laboratory of Structural Biology, and NINDS grant PO1 NS15654-14/15.

References

Abbott DH (1987) Behaviorally mediated suppression of reproduction in female primates. J Zool 213:455–470

Abrams RM, Ito M, Frisinger JE, Patlak CS, Pettigre KD, Kennedy C (1984) Local cerebral glucose utilization in fetal and neonatal sheep. Am J Physiol 246:R608–618

Amaral DG (1993) Morphological analyses of the brains of behaviorally characterized aged nonhuman primates. Neurobiol Aging 14:671–672

Andrews MW, Rosenblum LA (1993) Assessment of attachment in differentially reared infant monkeys (Macaca radiata): response to separation and a novel environment. J Comp Psychol 107: 84–90

Appel NM, Mitchell WM, Contrera JR, De Souza EB(1990) Effects of high dose fenfluramine treatment on monoamine uptake sites in rat brain: assessment using quantitative autoradiography. Synapse 6:33–44

Argen H, Mefford IV, Rudorfer MV, Linnoila M, Potter WA (1986) Interacting neurotransmitter systems: a non-experimental approach to the 5HIAA-HVA correlation in human CSF. J Psychiat Res 20:175–193

Berman CM (1992) Immature siblings and mother-infant relationships among free-ranging rhesus monkeys on Cayo Santiago. Anim Behav 44:247–258

Bernstein IS, Ruehlmann TE, Judge PG, Lindquist T, Weed JL (1991) Testosterone changes during the period of adolescence in male rhesus monkeys (Macaca mulatta). Am J Primat 24:29–38

Boothe R, Dobson V, Teller D (1985) Postnatal development of vision in human and non-human primates. Ann Rev Neurosci 8:495–545

Botchin MB, Kaplan JR, Manuck SB, Mann JJ (1993) Low versus high prolactin responders to fenfluramine challenge: markers of behavioral differences in adult male cynomologous macaques. Neuropsychopharmacology 9:93–99

Bourgeois JP (1993) Synaptogenesis in the prefrontal cortex of the macaques. In: de Boysson-Bardies B, de Schonen S, Jusczyk P, McNeilage P, Morton J (eds). Developmental neurocognition: speech and face processing in the first year of life. Dordrecht, Kluwer Academic Publisher, 31–39

Bourgeois JP, Goldman-Rakic PS, Rakic P (1985) Synaptogenesis in the prefrontal cortex: quantitative EM analysis in pre- and postnatal rhesus monkeys. Abstr Neurosci Soc 11:154.2

Bourgeois JP, Jastreboff PJ, Rakic P (1989) Synaptogenesis in visual cortex of normal and preterm monkeys: evidence for intrinsic regulation of synaptic overproduction. PNAS 86:4297–4301

Bourgeois JP, Goldman-Rakic PS, Rakic P (1994) Synaptogenesis in the prefrontal cortex of rhesus monkeys. Cerebral Cortex 4:78–96

Brammer GL, McGuire MT, Raleigh MJ (1987) Similarity of 5-HT2 receptor sites in dominant and subordinate vervet monkeys. Pharmacol Biochem Behav 27:701–795

Brand S, Rakic P (1984) Cytodifferentiation and synaptogenesis in the neostriatum of fetal and neonatal rhesus monkeys. Anat Embryol 169:21–34

Brothers L, Ring B (1993) Mesial temporal neurons in the macaque monkey with responses selective for aspects of social stimuli. Behav Brain Res 57:53–61

Brown GL, Linnoila MI (1990) CSF serotonin metabolite (5-HIAA) studies in depression, impulsivity and violence. J Clin Psychiat 51:31–41

Bryan GK, Riessen AH (1989) Deprived somatosensory-motor experience in stumptailed monkey neocortex: dendritic spine density and dendritic branching of layer IIIB pyramidal cells. J Comp Neurol 286:208–217

Castell R, Sackett G (1973) Motor behaviors of neonatal rhesus monkeys: measurement techniques and early development. Devel Psychobiol 6:191–202

Charney DS, Krystal JJ, Southwick CH (1990) Serotonin function in panic and generalized anxiety disorders. Psychiatric Ann 20:593–602

Cheney DL, Seyfarth RM (1983) Non-random dispersal in free-ranging vervet monkeys: social and genetic consequences. Am Nat 122:392–412

Cheney DL, Seyfarth RM (1990) How monkeys see the world. Chicago, Chicago University Press

Cheney DL, Seyfarth RM, Smuts B (1986) Social relationships and social cognition in non-human primates. Science 234:1361–1366

Chugani HT, Phelps ME (1986) Maturational changes in cerebral function in infants determined by [18]FDG positron emission tomography. Science 231:840–843

Chugani HT, Phelps ME, Mazziotta JC (1987) Positron emission tomography study of human brain functional development. Ann Neurol 22:487–497

Chugani HT, Hovda DA, Villablanca JR, Phelps ME, Xu W-F (1991) Metabolic maturation of the brain: a study of local cerebral glucose utilization in the developing cat. J Cer Blood Flow Metab 11:35–47

Clark AS, MacLusky NJ, Goldman-Rakic PS (1988) Androgen binding and metabolism in the cerebral cortex of the developing rhesus monkey. Endocrinology 134:932–940

Clarke AS, Wittwer DJ, Abbott DH, Schneider ML (1994) Long-term effects of prenatal stress on HPA axis activity in juvenile rhesus monkeys. Devel Psychobiol 27(5):257–269

Clarke DD, Sokoloff L (1994) Circulation and energy metabolism of the brain. In: Siegel GJ, Agranoff BW, Albers RW, Molinoff PB (eds) Basic neurochemistry. Vth Edition. Raven, New York, 645–680

Cloninger CR (1987) A unified biosocial theory of personality and its role in the development of anxiety states: a reply to commentaries. Psychiat Dev 6:83–120

Damasio H, Grabowski T, Frank R, Galaburda A, Damasio AR (1994) The return of Phineas Gage: Clues about the brain from the skull of a famous patient. Science 264:1102–1105

Damasio AR (1994) Descartes' error. Emotion, Reasons and the human brain. Grosset/Putnam, New York

Diamond A, Goldman-Rakic PS (1989) Comparison of human infants and rhesus monkeys on Piaget's AB task: evidence for dependence on dorsolateral prefrontal cortex. Exp Brain Res 74:24–40

Duffy CJ, Rakic P (1983) Differentiation of granule cell dendrites in the dentate gyrus of the rhesus monkey: a quantitative Golgi study. J Comp Neurol 214:224–237

Duffy TE, Cavazzutti M, Gregoire NM, Cruz NF, Kennedy C, Sokoloff L (1979) Regional cerebral glucose metabolism in newborn beagle dogs. Trans Am Soc Neurochem 10:171

Eckenhoff MF, Rakic P (1991) A quantitative analysis of synaptogenesis in the molecular layer of the dentate gyrus in the rhesus monkey. Dev Brain Res 64:129–135

Fairbanks LA (1993) Juvenile vervet monkeys: establishing relationships and practicing skills for the future. In: Pereira ME, Fairbanks (eds) Juvenile primates: Life History, Development and Behavior. Oxford Univ Press, pp 211–227

Fairbanks LA, McGuire MT (1988) Long-term effects of early mothering behavior on responsiveness to the environment in vervet monkeys. Dev Psychobiol 21:711–724

Fragazy DM, Adams-Curtis LE (1991) Generative aspects of manipulation in tufted capuchin monkeys (Cebus apella). J Comp Psychol 105:387–397

Friedman HR, Goldman-Rakic PS (1994) Coactivation of prefrontal cortex and inferior parietal cortex in working memory tasks revealed by 2DG functional mapping in the rhesus monkey. J Neurosci 14(5):2775–2788

Fuller RW (1992) Basic advances in serotonin pharmacology. J Clin Psychiat 53 (suppl):36–53

Fuster JM (1989) The prefrontal cortex. Raven Press, New York

Gibson KR (1991) Myelination and behavioral development: a comparative perspective on questions of neoteny, altriciality and intelligence. In: Gibson KR, Petersen AC (eds) Brain maturation and cognitive development: comparative and cross-cultural perspectives. New York, Aldine de Gruyter, 29–63

Goldman-Rakic PS (1988) Topography of cognition: parallel distributed networks in primate association cortex. Ann Rev Neurosci 11:137–156

Goldman-Rakic PS (1993) Neocortical memory cells and circuits. In: Andersen P, Hvalby O, Paulsen O, Hokfelt B (eds) Memory concepts: basic and clinical aspects. Amsterdam, Elsevier Science Publishers, pp 271–280

Goldman-Rakic PS, Brown RM (1982) Postnatal development of monoamine content and synthesis in the cerebral cortex of rhesus monkeys. Dev Brain Res 4:339–349

Gregoire N, Ponteir R, Salamon G (1981) Local cerebral glucose utilizations in the newborn brain. Eur Neurol 20:162–168

Greenough WT (1992) Induction of brain structure by experience: substrates for cognitive development. Minn Symp Child Psychol 24:155–200

Gunderson VM, Sackett GP (1984) Development of pattern recognition in infant pigtailed macaques (Macaca nemistrina). Dev Psychol 20:418–426

Gunderson VM, Yonas A, Sargent PL, Grant-Webster KS (1993) Infant macaque monkeys respond to pictorial depth. Psychol Sci 4(2):93–98

Harlow HF (1969) Age-mate or peer affectional system. Adv Study Behav 2:333–383

Higley JD, Hopkins WD, Thompson WW, Byrne EA, Hirsch RM, Suomi SJ (1992a) Peers as primary attachment sources in yearling rhesus monkeys (Macaca mulatta). Dev Psych 28(6):1163–1171

Higley JD, Mehlman PT, Taub DM, Higley SB, Suomi SJ, Linnoila M, Vickers JH (1992b) Cerbrospinal fluid monoamine and adrenal correlates of aggression in free-ranging rhesus monkeys. Arch Gen Psychiat 49:436–441

Higley JD, Thompson WT, Champoux M, Goldman M, Haser MR, Kraemer GW, Scanlan JM, Suomi SJ, Linnoila M (1993) Paternal and maternal genetic and environmental contributions to cerebrospinal fluid monoamine metabolites in Rhesus monkeys (*Macaca mulatta*). Arch Gen Psychiat 50:615–623

Insel TR, Winslow JT (1992) Neurobiology of obsessive compulsive disorder. Psychiat Clin North America 15(4):813–824

Isbell LA (1990) Sudden short-term increase in predation among vervet monkeys (Cercopithecus aethiops) due to leopard predation in Amboseli National Park, Kenya. Am J Primatol 21:41–52

Jacobs B, Scheibel AB (1993) A quantitative dendritic analysis of Wernicke's area in humans. I. Lifespan changes. J Comp Neurol 327:83–96

Kaplan JR, Botchin MB, Berard J, Manuck SB, Mann JJ (1995) Delayed dispersal and elevated monoaminergic activity in free-ranging rhesus monkeys. Am J Primatol, in press

Kennedy C, Sakurada O, Shinohara M, Miyaoka M (1982) Local cerebral glucose utilization in the newborn macaque monkey. Ann Neurol 12:333–340

King FA, Yarbrough CJ, Anderson DC, Gordon TP, Gould KG (1988) Primates. Science 240:1475–1482

Kraemer GW (1992) A psychobiological theory of attachment. Behav Brain Sci 15:493–541

Kraemer GW, Ebert MH, Schmidt DE, McKinney WT (1989) A longitudinal study of the effects of different social rearing conditions on cerebrospinal fluid norepinephrine and biogenic amine metabolites in rhesus monkeys. Neuropsychopharmacology 2:175–189

Lidow MS, Rakic P (1992) Scheduling of monoaminergic neurotransmitter receptor expression in the primate neocortex during postnatal development. Cereb Cortex 2:401–416

Lidow MS, Goldman-Rakic PS, Rakic P (1991) Synchronized overproduction of neurotransmitter receptors in diverse regions of the primate cerebral cortex. Proc Natl Acad Sci (USA) 88:10218–10221

McGuire MT, Raleigh MJ, Pollack DB (1994) Personality features in vervet monkeys: the effects of sex, age, social status, and group composition. Am J Primatol 33(1):1–14

Martin LJ, Spicer DM, Lewis MH, Gluck JP, Cork LC (1991) Social deprivation of infant rhesus monkeys alters the chemoarchitecture of the brain: I. Subcortical regions. J Neurosci 11:3334–3358

Mason WA, Long D, Mendoza S (1993) Temperament and mother-infant conflict in macaques: a transactional analysis. In: Mason WA, Mendoza SP (eds) Primate social conflict. New York, SUNY Press, 205–227

Meinecke DL, Rakic P (1992) Expression of GABA and GABA$_A$ receptors by neurons in the subplate zone in developing primate occipital cortex: evidence for transient local circuits. J Comp Neurol 317:91–101

Mori K, Schmidt K, Jay T, Palombo E, Nelson T, Lucignani G, Pettigrew K, Kennedy C, Sokoloff L (1990) Optimal duration of experimental period in measurement of local cerebral glucose utilization with the deoxyglucose method. J Neurochem 54:307–319

Nehlig A, Pereira De Vasconcelos A, Boyet S (1988) Quantitative autoradiographic measurement of local cerebral glucose utilization in freely moving rats during postnatal development. J Neurosci 8:2321–2333

O'Kusky R, Colonnier M (1982) Postnatal changes in the number of neurons and synapses in the visual cortex (area 17) of the macaque monkey: a stereological analysis in normal and monocularly deprived animals. J Comp Neurol 210:291–306

Peroutka SJ (1988) 5-hydroxytryptamine receptor subtypes. Ann Rev Neurosci 11:45–60

Pfaff DW (1982) Neurobiological mechanisms of sexual motivation. In: Pfaff DW (ed) The physiological mechanisms of motivation. New York, Springer-Verlag, 287–317

Phelps ME, Mazziota JC, Schelbert HR (1986) Positron emission tomography and autoradiography. New York, Raven Press

Plant TM (1988) Neuroendocrine basis of puberty in the monkey (Macaca mulatta). In: Martin L, Ganong W (eds) Frontiers in neuroendocrinology. Vol 19. New York: Raven Press Ltd, 215–238

Rakic P, Bourgeois P-P, Eckenhoff MF, Zecevic N, Goldman-Rakic PS (1986) Concurrent overproduction of synapses in diverse regions of the primate cerebral cortex. Science 232:232–235

Raleigh MJ, McGuire MT (1990) Social influences on endocrine function in male vervet monkeys. In: Ziegler TE, Bercovitch FB (eds) Socioendocrinology of primate reproduction. New York, Wiley-Liss Inc, 95–111

Raleigh MJ, McGuire MT (1991) Bidirectional relationships between tryptophan and social behavior in vervet monkeys. In: Schwarcz R, Young SN, Brown RR (eds) Kynurenine and serotonin pathways. New York, Plenum Press, 289–298

Raleigh MJ, McGuire MT (1994) Serotonin, aggression, and violence in vervet monkeys. In: Masters R, McGuire MT (eds) The neurotransmitter revolution: serotonin, social behavior and the law. Carbondale, IL, Southern Illinois University Press, 129–145

Raleigh MJ, McGuire MT, Brammer GL, Pollack DB, Yuwiler A (1991) Serotonergic mechanisms promote dominance acquisition in adult male vervet monkeys. Brain Res 559:181–190

Raleigh MJ, Brammer GL, McGuire MT, Pollack DB, Yuwiler A (1992) Individual differences in basal cisternal cerebrospinal fluid 5-HIAA and HVA in monkeys: the effects of gender, age, physical characteristics, and matrilineal influences. Neuropsychopharmacology 7(4):295–304

Rosenblum LA, Paully GS (1984) The effects of varying environmental demands on maternal and infant behavior. Child Devel 55:305–314

Ruppenthal G, Sackett GP (1992) A guide to the care, feeding, and evaluation of infant monkeys. Seattle, University of Washington Press

Sanders-Bush E (1988) The serotonin receptors. Clifton NJ, Humana Press

Sapolsky RM (1990) Adrenocortical function, social rank, and personality among wild baboons. Biol Psychiat 28:862–878

Schneider ML (1992) Delayed object permanence development in prenatally stressed rhesus monkey infants (Macaca mulatta). Occupat Ther J Res 12(2):96–110

Shaw C, Cameron L, March D, Cynader M, Zielinski B, Hendrickson A (1991) Pre- and postnatal development of GABA receptors in Macaca monkey visual cortex. J Neurosci 11:3943–3959

Shelton SE, Kalin NH, Gluck JP, Kerestutry MF, Schneider VA, Lewis MH (1988) Effect of age on cisternal cerebrospinal fluid concentrations of monoamine metabolites in nonhuman primates. Neurochem Int 13:353–357

Simpson MJA, Howe S (1988) Group and matriline differences in the behavior of rhesus monkey infants. Anim Behav 34:444–459

Sokoloff L, Reivich M, Kennedy C, Des Rosiers MH, Patlak CS, Pettigrew KD, Sakurada O, Shinohara M (1977) The (^{14}C) deoxyglucose method for the measurement of local cerebral glucose utilization: theory, procedure, and normal values in the conscious and anesthetized albino rat. J Neurochem 28:897–916

Struhsaker TT (1971) Social behavior of mother and infant vervet monkeys (Cercopithecus aethiops). Anim Behav 19:233–250

Suomi SJ (1991) Uptight and laid-back monkeys: individual differences in the response to social challenges. In: Brauth SE, Hall WS, Dooling RJ (eds) Plasticity of development. Cambridge, Massachusetts, MIT Press, 27–56

Virkkunen M, Rawlings R, Tokola T, Poland RE, Guidotti A, Nemeroff C, Bissette G, Kalogeras K, Karonen S, Linnoila M (1994) CSF biochemistries, glucose metabolism, and diurnal activity rhythms in alcoholic,violent offenders, fire setters, and healthy volunteers. Arch Gen Psychiat 51:20–27

Wagner J, Peroutka SJ (1990) Neurochemistry and neurotoxicity of substituted amphetamines. Neuropsychopharmacology 3:219–220

Westergaard GC (1993) Development of combinatorial manipulation in infant baboons (Papio cynocephalus anubis). J Comp Psychol 107(91):34–38

Wenk GL, Pierce DJ, Struble RG, Price DL, Cork LC (1989) Age-related changes in multiple neurotransmitter systems in the monkey brain. Neurobiol Aging 10:11–19

Williams SM, Goldman-Rakic PS (1993) Characterization of the dopaminergic innervation of the primate frontal cortex using a dopamine-specific antibody. Cerebral Cortex 3:199–222

Wilson MA, Molliver ME (1991) The organization of serotonergic projections to cerebral cortex in primates: retrograde transport studies. Neuroscience 44(3):555–570

Young SN, Teff KL (1989) Trytophan availability, 5-HT synthesis, and 5-HT function. Prog Neuropsychopharm Biol Psychiatr 13:373–379

Zecevic N, Rakic P (1991) Synaptogenesis in the primary somatosensory cortex of the Macaque rhesus during fetal and postnatal life. Cerebral Cortex 1:510–523

Zecevic N, Bourgeois JP, Rakic P (1989) Changes in synaptic density in motor cortex of rhesus monkey during fetal and postnatal life. Dev Brain Res 50:11–32

Neural Basis of Decision in Perception and in the Control of Movement

A. Berthoz

It is a very rare privilege for a physiologist to be allowed to speculate without providing the experimental proofs of his statements. Although admittedly dangerous, this type of exercise is necessary for the development of our discipline. The present paper will take the form of a review of experimental and theoretical work. In addition, it will try to propose very preliminary thoughts on and around the question of the neural basis of decision.

In this paper I will first mention a theory of how the brain generates and controls sensory motor processes, because I believe that one cannot study the neural basis of decision without an explicit hypothesis concerning the mechanisms of brain operations. I will then present a few examples concerning decisions related to motion perception, and finally I will give a more detailed description of how I believe decisions are made in a particular motor behaviour: the control of gaze and visual exploration.

Firstly I would like to suggest that decision is not a new discovery of the primate and human brain. The tendency to attribute a prominent role in decision processes to the prefrontal cortex is an honourable attempt to account for complex decision processes in the social life of humans. It is now clear that the frontal and prefrontal cortex play an essential role in the processes of planning, prediction, memory and more generally what has been called "theories of mind." namely the capacity to predict other people's on animals intention. But in looking for fundamental neural mechanisms underlying decisions, it may be interesting to also build a theory including other levels of the central nervous system. In particular it is interesting to study how decisions are made in perception and action and not only in social life. Higher cognitive functions are derived from the necessity to plan future action from past experiences and make decisions about action. This implies that spatial cognition is as or even more important to study than language.

Let us rapidly review some arguments to show that decision is present even in very primitive neural systems. The key neurone for escape behaviour in the squid, in a sense, represents the integration of all sensory cues "meaning danger." Embodied in its morphology and intrinsic properties (Llinas 1974), this primitive cell has all the elements necessary for a "decision." It will fire a spike only when a

Laboratoire de Physiologie de la Perception et de l'Action, Collège de France-CNRS, UMR 9950, Paris, France

A.R. Damasio et al. (Eds.)
Neurobiology of Decision-Making
© Springer-Verlag Berlin Heidelberg 1996

configuration (a combination of simultaneously occurring events) of sensory cues in the environment means "danger" for the animal, if conflicting cues are presented the animal will have to make a decision.

It should also be remembered that decision-making is a fundamental property of the neural systems underlying prey-predator related behaviour. Ewert and his colleagues (see for instance Matsumoto et al. 1991) has beautifully shown that, although the toad will produce a prey catching behaviour to a target that is elongated and whose velocity is aligned with its greater length, it will, by contrast, trigger an escape reaction if the target has the shape of a large pattern with no specific rectangular shape. Ewert has shown that the "decision" to trigger either type of behaviour is made by a very simple neural mechanism: specialised neurons detect the main features of the targets as described above and then they mutually inhibit each other. This mechanism is adaptable and can be modified by training.

Decisions in higher organisms may in fact be produced by mechanisms that appeared earlier during evolution and have been used for the control of sensory motor processes. If this is the case, the problem of the "embodiment" of decision becomes an ill-posed problem. Our field is dominated by models derived from either logic or computer science that implicitly use the "computer metaphor." The discovery by Damasio and his colleagues (1991, 1994) that galvanic skin response is associated with complex choices then appears as a surprise in this hypothetical framework, and his discussion of an "embodiment" of higher cognitive functions, synthesised in his book, *Descartes' error*, is an elegant attempt to return to a more biological description of the relations between the brain and the body.

The Brain as a Simulator

Let us now examine a theory of brain function to set a frame for discussions. We have proposed (Droulez et al. 1985; Berthoz et al. 1989) the following ideas concerning brain function.

During an action, sensory motor processes are operating through two parallel modes. One mode consists of sensory motor loops linking the sensors to the central nervous system and the effectors. These sensory motor loops work as conservative processes like cybernetic loops. They are continuous, have properties similar to servomechanisms, deal with sensory signals that are transformed into motor commands through the construction of motor errors and are regulated by feed-back or feed-forward mechanism. They operate on a repertoire of motor synergies that generate a set of motor primitives. In this mode the brain operates as a *controller*.

But we have also proposed the idea that, in paralled with this controller, higher central loops that have increasingly gained complexity during evolution operate on another mode that we have called a projective process. In this mode, signals are processed in internal loops having no direct link with sensors. The operations are discontinuous (they can be triggered in an intermittent fashion), and they occur on neural maps in which the important parameters are the topological relations between the neurones. This mode produces predictions of future states and it preselects strategies (which themselves are combinations of synergies and combinations of expected states of sensors). In this mode the brain works as a modular *simulator*.

At present no definite proof has been obtained to demonstrate the validity of this model. However, some emphasis has been recently placed on the importance of self-sustained inner loops, like for example the possible functional role of basal ganglia-thalamo-cortical loops (Alexander et al. 1986). Within these loops it has been proposed that 40 Hz oscillations (Llinas 1988) would sustain an endogenous activity which would be due to intrinsic oscillatory properties of some thalamic neurons. Thus the brain could use this self sustained activity without external stimuli to evolve representations of space and movement (as occurs during dreams). The importance of this model for the study of the neural basis of decision is that if this model is correct, then decisions are basic operations of the projective system. There must, of course, be a very important difference between the elementary decision of the toad performing a choice between catching and avoiding reaction and higher cognitive decisions using internal simulations in reentrant loops.

These facts however support our proposal (Berthoz 1993) that the brain is not a machine responds to external stimuli but a machine that formulates hypotheses based upon internally generated simulations of action. The decision to make one movement rather than another is, therefore, an essential part of the normal function of sensory-motor systems. It also involves not only the prefrontal cortex but many different levels that participate in decisions at multiple degrees of complexity with respect to the choice of the effectors, the choice of the motor repertoire, the relations with the context, the integration of memories of past episodes, etc . . .

Seen from this point of view, the existence of "somatic events" associated with decisions does not in any sense mean that these somatic events are the "markers" of what Premack (1993) would call the "value" of previously made decisions. These somatic events could indicate that, when a subject is making a decision, he is truly "simulating" the consequences of his decisions and therefore that this simulation includes the predicted vegetative consequences of the simulated sequence of behaviours.

Perception Is a Decision

In the case of perception, decision is necessary for several reasons, including, for example, the case of ambiguous sensory signals or for the selection of relevant sensory cues and their relation with action. If perception is closely linked to action, it can no longer be a simple process of passive transformation from sensory transducer activity into central representations; the control of action requires predictive mechanisms which in turn require a preselection of relevant sensory information and what I would like to call "pre-perceptions:" going down a slope when skiing is too fast for any continuous control of movement. The brain has to predict the expected state of those sensory cues which are relevant for each phase of the movements and only sample their state intermittently. A number of experimental results demonstrate this preselection of sensory cues during natural movements. This preselection has been demonstrated in the cases of locomotion or of complex natural hand movements by Lacquaniti (Lacquaniti 1989, 1992; see also reviews in Berthoz 1993a), who has recently shown that the mechanical impact of catching a ball is internally simulated and predicted probably using an internal model of the limb. These models of body parts may very well be generated by oscillations that occur in newborn animals and adjust the presynaptic of central neural circuits to the mechanical properties of the limbs (Llinas et al. 1988).

The selection of sensory cues is accomplished by the efferent gating of sensory inputs (for instance by presynaptic inhibition) but also by modulation of sensory inputs by corollary signals ("efferenzcopy"). The gamma system of the neuromuscular spindles is a beautiful example of an "outflow mechanism" that allows modulation of sensory inputs at the very level of the receptor. In general, efferent control of receptors should be understood not only as cybernetics theories view it – a way to perform gain control of sensors – but also as a mechanism of anticipation, of selection. It is well known that sensory signals in the spinal cord are influenced at the first central synapse by motor signals related to intended action. This is true for the vestibular nuclear neurones that are modulated by gaze signals (Berthoz et al. 1989), or for thalamic relay neurones in the visual pathways like the lateral ventral geniculate nucleus, or for the intra-laminar nucleus whose activity is modulated by eye movements (Magnin et al. 1974). It is also true for the pathways mediating tactile sensitivity, in which cells firing in response to a tactile stimulus are conditional to an active exploration. Mistlin and Perret (1990) have shown that transmission of sensory signals to the cortex is conditional to an active exploration, and one may remember the paper by Perl many years ago showing tactile sensory gating in the rat.

Perception does not, therefore, concern only the reconstruction of the external world by successive transformation and binding of sensory cues in the "space" of the sensors. It also probably is made of decision processes *matching* external configurations of features with an internally predetermined or acquired *repertoire* of sensory or motor patterns.

Self-Motion Perception: A Decision Process?

We shall now review some examples to show the remarkable flexibility of perception which demonstrate that decision is indeed an intrinsic part of active perception or that perception *IS* a decision. I will not borrow these examples from the classical case of vision, although visual perception provides infinite sources to demonstrate this idea. I will consider examples that pertain to the fact that the brain has to solve problems of "configurations of sensory inputs" in the sense of Gibson (1966).

Let us consider the particular case of self-motion perception. It is well known that visual, vestibular and tactile cues contribute to the perception of body motion. Their signals have to be blended into a coherent construct. Any discongruence between the various sensory cues induces either illusory movements or disorientation and vertigo. Lackner and his colleagues have studied this problem extensively (Lackner 1988; Lackner and Levine 1979). Let us consider the case of a subject who is lying in a machine that exposes him to what has been called a "Barbecue spit" stimulus. In this experiment the subject is subjected, in total darkness, to rotation around an earth-horizontal axis. The only sensors that detect his movement are the vestibular organs and the tactile receptors. The subjective perception induced in this condition is that of a rotation around an horizontal axis. However, if a gentle push is exerted on the head or the buttocks, the subject will suddenly feel that he is rotating around a completely different axis. His percept is therefore driven by the pressure on the skin, which is used by the brain as a cue for deciding where the centre and the axis of rotation are.

I consider that this sudden shift in perception is a real decision taken by the brain according to probable or memorised experiences. The brain performs a real "bet" in favour of one interpretation or another. I think that it is a serious error to call these percepts "illusions." On the contrary, I believe that these interpretations are solutions: *"Illusions are solutions and perceptual decisions which are taken by the brain when it is faced with discongruent sensory inputs."*

Another example is provided by the perception of self-motion induced by moving visual fields. This phenomenon is called "vection." Since the early studies by Mach (1967) we know that vision is a basic sensor for the perception of self-motion. The psychophysical properties of vection have been extensively studied by several authors in recent years (Dichgans and Brandt 1978; Berthoz et al. 1975; Sauvan and Bonnet 1993; Brandt et al. 1973; Büttner and Henn 1981; de Graaf et al. 1990). The intensity of vection is dependent upon the size of the visual field, the spatial and temporal frequency of the visual patterns, and the foreground and background relations. Even very small visual stimuli can induce vection if they are presented in the proper environmental context.

However, one problem is still unsolved: when the visual world moves, the brain can interpret this movement as either a movement of the world or as a movement of the body in a stable environment. The above-mentioned studies indicate what parameters may determine a "decision" in favour of the former or the latter interpretation. However, we still do not know the exact mechanisms the brain uses to finally put the emphasis on one of these two interpretations, Information about self-motion is built into the vestibular nucleus by convergent vestibular, visual and proprioceptive signals. But the cortical pathways and mechanisms responsible for the comparison of purely visual motion and self motion are not known.

However, we have made interesting progress in recent years. In particular, a very important discovery was made by Grüsser and his colleagues (1982, 1990a,b). They found an area in the temporal cortex, located in the vicinity of the insula, that contains neurones activated by vestibular, visual and proprioceptive signals and that codes head movement in space during rotations. This structure receives projections from the vestibular nuclei through the sensory thalamus and in turn projects to various areas in the cortex. Several cortical areas in the monkey receive these vestibular signals: area 7a, Area 2V and 3a, area T3, and the cingulate gyrus. From these structures, or in some of them, the signals about visual world motion carried through the occipital pathways and those ascending through the vestibular system can be compared. But we do not know yet how the "decision" is made.

The preceding example concerns a problem of perceptual decision. We shall now consider some examples of perceptuo-motor decisions. We know of many occasions in which the brain cannot make perceptuo-motor decisions. A very spectacular example is provided by the "landing freeze" or the "Y crossroad freeze" syndrome. While landing an aircraft, some pilots who are suddenly faced with a difficult decision are totally paralysed for a few seconds, and the co-pilot has to take over to avoid a catastrophe. The same freeze happens to automobile drivers when they are faced with a Y-type crossroad in which the decision to go left or right is somehow equiprobable. They generally keep going straight!

This paralysis probably comes from the sudden incapacity to decide between two alternatives. Several theories can be proposed to explain this blockage of behaviour:

A sensory theory: the subject analyses the two sensory configurations of cues in series but cannot elaborate a comparison scale (probably not adequate).

A motor theory: from sensory cues the subject knows the decision that he should make depending upon his own goals, but does not generate the adequate motor act (probably not adequate either).

A matching theory: the subject cannot match the sensory cues to their existing motor repertoire of behaviour. The difficulty lies in the relationship between the interpretation of sensory information and the motor act.

A prediction theory: the subject can very well evaluate the two situations and the corresponding motor responses, but he fails to predict the consequences of each action and has, therefore, no criteria to anticipate upon the value of each solution.

A matching to memory theory: the subject can evaluate the consequences of his action. If the action involves other animals or humans, he can even build a "theory of mind" of the partner, but he cannot compare the prediction to previous experience, either because of the novelty of the situation or because of threatening memories. In this latter case he is "negatively marked," in the sense of Damasio.

A behaviour selection theory: the subject can evaluate the condition well, predicts the consequences of each action, compares with previous memories and attaches a sign to the potential choice. But he cannot simulate internally this new choice because he cannot select the levels at which action is internally simulated. The main problem is, therefore, a problem of selective blockage of execution during the internal simulation of the predicted action. This could be because some ambiguities arise as to the systems that have to be released and those that have to be inhibited or because of lack of time for an adequate internal simulation without execution. The subject, therefore, cannot establish an adequate set of predicted sensory cues on which to base his behaviour and just inhibits behaviour. In other words the brain has no time to build a coherent hypothesis in its inner loops.

In the view of Damasio (1994) the reduction of degrees of freedom for a decision is made by the evocation of somatic markers that give colour to categories of solutions. This is indeed one way to eliminate categories of solutions. Another way is to consider that the brain does not have time for such comparisons and that rapid decisions are made by a mechanism opposite to that proposed by Damasio (1994). In our view the association of gut feelings to decisions is the consequence of internal simulations that create discongruence in internal models of the body. The brain is a matching machine and a simulator of action, not a "representational" machine, not a computer which calculates solutions and gives them some "value." The brain is essentially a comparer. Activity in inner reentrant loops simulates, or emulates, a repertoire of behaviours that has to be permanently inhibited. A decision to make something is, therefore, essentially the decision not to make all the others. A very good example of this idea is modern theories of depression, which have revealed that depressed people keep rehearsing undecidable situations.

A Hierarchical Gating Theory of Decision on Motor Control

The brain is, therefore, a simulator that has the essential property of predicting the future from past or current experience. Experimental proofs of this simulator nature have come recently from data showing that the same structures are activated during imagined and executed movements, as we will see below. In my opinion a very fundamental, dynamic neural mechanism that allows decision to be made is gating by cascades of synaptic inhibition. I have chosen to give examples to support this theory that are taken from the neural organisation of gaze orienting. For instance, "anti-saccade" paradigms, or the organisation of complex saccadic sequences, may represent an interesting model for the study of the neural basis of motor decision.

One of the most important elements of the repertoire of motor behaviour is visual exploration. This fundamental behaviour is performed by a very simple movement: eye saccades. But this apparently simple movement is in fact an extremely interesting model for the study of decision. If, as Yarbus first did (Yarbus 1967), we ask a subject to look at a lady's face and pay attention to whether this lady is rich or is sad, or if now we ask the subject to look at a landscape and analyse the scene to find if there are animals or trees, or if the sky is clear, the "scan-path" of saccades will be different in these different cases. Complex cognitive decisions have to be made in order to scan a part of the face or the scene. Saccades are, therefore, an element of the motor repertoire with which we can think about the neural basis of decisions.

The study of the neural mechanisms of eye saccades has made extraordinary progress in the last decade due to the convergence of neurobiology, modelling

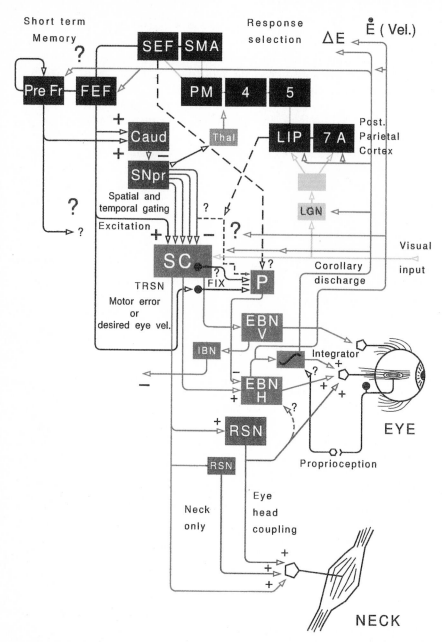

Fig. 1. Schematic representation of the main levels that underlie the production of orienting eye and head movements. The purpose of this diagram is not to show the detailed neuronal circuits that underlie saccade or head movement generation but to support the idea that the decision to make an orienting movement with the eye or with the head, or both, is taken through a hierarchy of parallell excitatory and inhibitory mechanisms. The eye saccade is produced by excitatory burst neurone (EBN) located in the pontine and mesencephalic reticular formation. EBN-V and EBN-H indicate the immediate premotor burst neurones that provide the velocity gaze signals to the eye. The saccadic integrator

neuroanatomy, and neuropsychology. I will present in this paper a review of the mechanisms that control eye saccades from a very special point of view. My purpose here is not to give a detailed account of saccadic neuronal mechanisms step by step but to give a general overview of how I think the saccadic system is organised in order to propose a theory concerning decision-making in movement control.

I believe that non-reflexive eye saccades are produced by neural mechanisms that involve several parallel loops that are arranged in cascade in such a way that excitatory processes are inhibited at several levels. This arrangement allows an internal simulation of eye movement even in the absence of overt saccades. Such a multilevel inhibition of the process allows spatial and temporal selection and internal predictions that are the mechanisms that give an overt impression of a unified decision. In this process the prefrontal cortex, although probably important in some higher level decisions, is only one of the areas in which decision occurs. The "embodiment" of decisions is related to the fundamentally "distributed" nature of the decision process and may be not only to some mysterious "somatic marking."

But let us consider the way saccades are produced, making a "bottom-up" description. The main ideas concerning this question are summarised on the schema drawn on Figure 1.

---

is indicated by the symbol (∫) only for EBN-H. Note that the information on eye displacement (ΔE) and eye velocity (Ė) is sent through ascending pathways as a corollary discharge of the premotor elements. The discharge of EBN-H is under the inhibitory control of the pause neurones (P), which constitute a temporal gating device located at the immediate premotor level. Therefore the cortical and collicular circuits can be activated but the execution of the saccade is controlled by this premotor lock. Pause neurones are themselves inhibited, probably by two parallel routes, one descending directly from the frontal eye fields (FEF) and the second descending from the rostral pole of the superior colliculus (in the monkey). However, the exact mechanism underlying fixation is not known. A second level is represented by the superior colliculus (SC), which mediates visually guided saccades and also some saccades from memory. Intermediate layers of the SC contain tecto-reticulo-spinal neurones (TRSNs), which project to the pontine and mesencephalic saccade generators. Saccade initiation by these neurones is only possible if the tonic inhibition exerted by the substantia nigra pars reticulata (SNpr) on the SC map is suppressed. The SNpr exerts a spatial and temporal selection on this map. The SNpr is itself under inhibitory control from the caudate nucleus (Caud). In addition to this inhibitory cascade, a second one that is not shown here has been found to be mediated through the sub-thalamic nucleus.

This mechanism is probably fundamental for "selective attention," and this diagram supports a "motor theory" of selective attention.

The diagram also shows that the basal ganglia structures involved in orienting movement generation are part of cortico-thalamo-basal ganglia loops, which probably allow internal simulation of some aspects of the movement.

Cortical structures involved in eye movement generation are indicated schematically. Several structures probably involved in the internal mechanisms responsible for saccade generation and control are not shown (cingulate cortex, pulvinar, etc . . .). *SEF*, supplementary eye field; *SMA*, supplementary motor area; *PM*, premotor cortex; *PreFr*, prefrontal cortex; *LIP*, lateral inferior parietal lobule; *LGN*, lateral geniculate nucleus; *FIX*, fixation; *IBN*, inhibitory burst neuron; *RSN*, reticulo-spinal neuron

Decision by Premotor Temporal Gating

The saccade is produced by a pulse step discharge of extraocular motoneurones. This discharge is induced by a single premotor mechanism (see reviews in Fuchs et al. 1985; Yoshida et al. 1982; Kaneko et al. 1981) that is the discharge of "excitatory burst neurones" (EBNs) and their inhibitory counterparts, "inhibitory burst neurones" (IBNs), located in the pontine reticular formation for horizontal saccades and in the mesencephalic reticular formation for vertical saccades. The EBNs activate an integrator circuit whose exact nature is yet unknown but which certainly involves a structure called the nucleus prepositus hypoglossi, whose function in eye movement control was discovered by Baker and Berthoz (1975). It is the combination of the burst produced by the EBNs and the tonic component of the tonic (T) premotor neurones that produces the adequate motor discharge of the extraocular motoneurones during a saccaed. It is important to note that the final common premotor interneurones for saccades are the EBNs. They receive descending activation from neurones located in the intermediate layers of the superior colliculus (Moschkovakis et al. 1988a,b), which may be either direct or through local, so-called long lead bursters.

A second group of neurones that controls ocular motoneurones during saccades are reticulo-spinal neurones (RSNs), whose soma are located in the reticular formation surrounding the abducens nucleus. These neurones have been studied by Grantyn and Berthoz (1987a,b). Some of them project to both the abducens nucleus and to the spinal cord and therefore subserve the ipsilateral orienting synergy of the eye and the head during orienting movements. They are eye-head coupling neurones. Others only project to the neck and produce phasic eye-head movements.

The important point for the present set of ideas is that this immediate premotor machinery is under the control of a locking neuronal device called the "pause neurones" (Curthoys et al. 1984). These neurones are located in the midline of the reticular formation rostrally to the abducens nucleus. They discharge tonically and are inhibitory in nature. They inhibit the EBNs and possibly the RSNs.

The first point I want to make here that is relevant to the problem of the neural basis of decisions is that the whole brain can activate the neuronal centres involved in the production of saccades, but if the pause neurones continue to fire, the saccade will not be executed because of the inhibitory gating by pause neurones at this immediate premotor level. We have here a mechanism that can allow the brain to internally stimulate an orienting of gaze without execution. The decision to make a saccade can be implemented by the release from premotor inhibitory gating. It should also be noted that the RSNs are under the control of both the cortex and the cerebellum (whose output is itself inhibitory), and that a cascade of inhibitory gating mechanisms may therefore be involved at this premotor level.

Decision by Spatial and Temporal Gating on Retinotopic Maps of the Superior Colliculus

We shall now turn to the next level at which decisions can be made. The intermediate layers of the superior colliculus contain efferent neurones, called tecto-reticulo-spinal neurones (TRSNs), that project to the brain stem and spinal cord and are premotor during saccadic eye movements. Several kinds of neurones have been described by Moshkovakis et al. (1988a,b) in this category, which differ by their somatic or axonal characteristics and also by their physiological properties. The exact mechanism of their contribution to the generation of saccades is still controversial, but a consensus has been reached that at least some of these neurones project to the brain stem and constitute the input to the EBNs and RSNs involved in the production of the saccade. Each of them constitutes a motor vector (Glimcher and Sparks 1992) in the sense that the geometry of the saccade that will be triggered by any neurone is determined by the axonal connectivity of the TRSNs in the brain stem and/or mesencephalic saccade generators (Grantyn and Berthoz 1985, 1987; Grantyn and Grantyn 1982). Geometry is therefore coded by axonal geometry. The remarkable property which I would like to stress is that these neurones are organised in a retinotopic map that is in register with the superficial layers of the superior colliculus. This motor map is under the inhibitory control of the substantia nigra (SN; Deniau and Chevalier 1981; Hikosaka and Wurtz 1983). In addition, Deniau and Chevalier have shown that the projection from the SN to the superior colliculus is very precisely organised. It has therefore been suggested that the SN exerts both a *temporal* and a *spatial* selection of the triggering and production of the saccade by SC neurones.

At the level of the SC, what we may call a spatio-temporal decision is elaborated which allows "selective attention" to be shifted to a given zone of space. We therefore discover a second level of gating of the orienting mechanisms.

Inhibitory Control of the SN Spatio-Temporal Selection by the Striatum

The other interesting example about the essential role of inhibitory mechanisms in saccade selection is provided by an inhibitory action of caudate neurones which was discovered and documented by Hikosaka and colleagues (Hikosaka et al. 1989a,b,c; 1993). A saccade can only be triggered if caudate neurones (themselves probably activated by frontal eye field neurones) inhibit SN neurones that, in turn, induce a disinhibition of SC neurones, which themselves excite EBNs if inhibitory pause neurones are inhibited. It has been shown that caudate neurones fire during memorised saccades and are probably involved in cognitive control of saccade initiation.

Therefore, we have another fine cascade of inhibitory mechanisms that may play a role in the decision processes of saccade planning. This very exquisite organisation is even more subtle than *one may think from what precedes*. Recent discoveries have shown that, paralleling this "selection by suppression" mechanism involving the caudate and SN, a second cascade of inhibitions and excitations produces a "selection by facilitation." This pathway, which goes through the subthalamic nucleus, may be important.

Inner Loops and Decision

In the introduction we reminded the reader of our previous theoretical proposal of "inner loops contributing to a projective mode of movement control." This part of our theory has recently obtained some support from the discovery of the potential important functional role of such circuits as the basal ganglia-thalamo-cortical loops. This suggests that saccades that are not produced by simple sequences along sensory to motor circuits but, as discussed above that "internal circuits" such as the basal ganglia-thalamo-cortical loops (Alexander et al. 1986) that are organised in modular loops related to several motor or behavioural functions and, as far as the "oculomotor loop" is concerned, probably play a fundamental role in the elaboration of oculomotor strategies. This concept of inner loops in which activity can be sustained also provides a new view concerning the way decision processes can be made.

The interesting contribution to our theory brought about by Hikosaka is that he has also proposed a theoretical circuit by which reward can influence the basal ganglia-thalamo-cortical loop involved in the regulation and selection of saccades. In his view the basal ganglia act as co-ordinators for the mutual interplay between the various cortical areas involved in the elaboration of a motor strategy. These areas would be functionally connected by reward-based learning. The outputs from these independent cortical areas would converge on the basal ganglia at the beginning of the learning. During learning, an association between the motor convergence and the reward signals coming from the limbic system would select at the level of the basal ganglia only those combinations of cortical inputs leading to reward.

This suggestion of a role in learning selective combinations of signals could, of course, be a property of structures others than the basal ganglia. The main point to be retained here in relation to the problem of the neural basis of decision is that the frontal and prefrontal cortex may not be the only structures involved in decision-making, at least in the domain of visuo-motor behaviour. It certainly involves several levels of gating from the immediate premotor levels to the basal ganglia thalamo-cortical circuits.

Cortical Selection Mechanisms

In the previous sections we insisted upon the possible role of subcortical mechanisms in decision processes to contrast with current trends that place the emphasis on the prefrontal cortex. However, it is clear that cortical structures also play a basic role in selection of saccades. Recent studies in humans (Gaymard et al. 1990,

1993; Pierrot-Deseilligny et al. 1991, 1993) have shown that the supplementary motor area (SMA), or more precisely the supplementary eye field (SEF), is probably essential for the organisation of sequences of saccades. Studies using positron emission tomography (Berthoz et al. 1992) have shown the activation of the SMA, frontal eye field and cingulate cortex during voluntary, self-initiated saccades, and of the same structures plus the parietal cortex and the prefrontal cortex during sequences of memorised saccades.

The detailed neuronal mechanisms involved in these selection processes are not known, but I would like to predict that, here again, in addition to excitatory mechanisms, inhibition will be a major component of the selection.

The prefrontal cortex should, of course, be considered as a major component of cognitively driven decisions in visuo-motor exploration. This is suggested by a number of results on animals and humans. The prefrontal cortex is involved in working memory. The initial neurophysiological evidence comes from single unit data from Funahashi and his colleagues (1989, 1993a,b), who discovered three principal kinds of neurones: 1) neurones that register the stimulus to be recalled; 2) neurones that retain the information on line; and 3) neurones that use the information to guide the appropriate response in direction and timing. In addition, a partial lesion of the dorsolateral prefrontal cortex in one hemisphere can disrupt the performance in an oculomotor delayed response task, particularly under circumstances of memory guidance. The same lesion has little effect when the eye movement is guided by external cues. Therefore the prefrontal cortex may not only be involved in visual representational memory but also in the capacity to select proper events. Data from Joseph and Barone (1987) and more recently by Boussaoud et al. (1993; Boussaoud and Wise 1993), indeed point in this direction.

Guitton et al. (1985) showed that patients with prefrontal lesions have deficits in the performance of the "anti-saccade task." In this task the subject is asked to make a saccade in the opposite direction to the location of the visual target, therefore combining a "no-go" instruction and a decision to go in the opposite direction. Since this pioneering experiment, several other studies have indicated the role of the frontal and prefrontal cortex in complex decision processes of saccade generation. Patients with frontal lobe lesions show impairment in the predictive aspects of saccade generation (Keating 1991). In addition, schizophrenic patients have been shown to have deficits in anti-saccade tasks and in delayed oculomotor tasks (Goldman-Rakic 1994; Park and Holzman 1992) and high levels of "distractability" (Krappmann et al., submitted for publication). This may indicate a lack of capacity to select and decide for a motor strategy. More generally, the so-called "no-go" paradigm may be an interesting one to understand some of the basic mechanisms underlying decision.

The involvement of the prefrontal cortex in decision processes cannot be separated from other neural centres involved in the inner loops along which spatial perception and movement control are simulated. For instance, as mentioned above, a recent PET study has revealed that, during the execution of internally generated sequences of memorised saccades, the parietal cortex, which was not activated by simple volontary saccades in the dark, is activated together with the prefrontal cortex, as if the visual areas or the parietal cortex would be activated to produce an internal replay of the sequences of visual targets.

In addition the data we have obtained suggest that the cingulate cortex is involved in the organisation or in the control of internally generated saccades. Several recent results obtained with brain imaging techniques either in the monkey or in man have provided new evidence that the several sub-parts of the cingulate are involved either in the post-saccadic adjustments, or in internally generated movements (Frith et al. 1991), or in cognitive tasks involving internally taken perceptual decisions. We could therefore suppose that the cingulate cortex is an essential station of the structures involved in "internal loops" in which movement or action are simulated, either during or in the absence of execution. However, more detailed experimental work is necessary to understand the role of the various parts of the cingulate cortex.

A last point should be added to these remarks. According to our theory of internal simulation of movement, short-term memory processes are involved in the internal simulation accompanying decision. One has therefore to postulate that the hippocampus is involved in the internally produced sequences of memorised saccades. Recent data from Pierrot-Deseilligny et al. (submitted for publication) seem to confirm this proposal.

Do Imagined Movements Utilise
the Same Structures as Executed Movements

According to our theory the same central neural networks should be involved in both imagined and executed movements. Motor imagery would not be a special process but only the manifestation of the normal internal simulation that accompanies the planning and execution of movements. To test this hypothesis we conducted an experiment (Lang et al. 1994) in which subjects were asked to produce saccades either imagined or really executed. This work lead to the conclusion (Fig. 2) that the SMA, FEF and cingulate cortex were activated during this task and that apparently the same parts of these structures were active during both the self paced executed saccades and the imagined saccades. This result agrees with the work by Decety et al. (1994; Decety and Michel 1989) on imagined movements. However, the precision of PET does not allow us to exclude the possibility that discrete areas within these regions, or even different types of neurones, are activated during these different tasks. In fact, only experimental results on monkey neurones will settle the question.

The activity in the structures involved in the production of saccades during imagined saccades also supports the idea that attention shifts share the same neuronal mechansims as orienting movements. This similarity between the mechanisms of attention and motor imagery was suggested by Posner et al. (1984) and was recently also promoted by Rizzolatti, who proposed a motor theory of attention (see review in Rizzolatti and Camarda 1987)

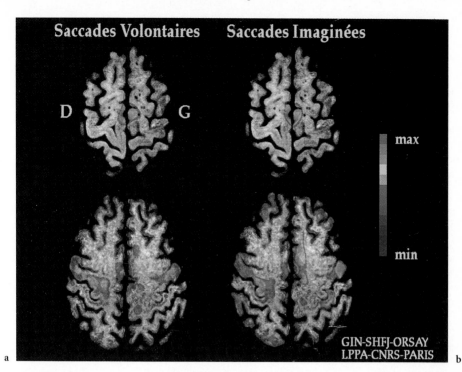

Saccades Volontaires   Saccades Imaginées

D   G

max

min

GIN-SHFJ-ORSAY
LPPA-CNRS-PARIS

a   b

Fig. 2. Are the same structures activated during imagined and executed movements? Positron emission tomography picture of the CBF activation map of cortical sites during both executed (**a**) and imagined (**b**) voluntary saccades. The maps were obtained at two different brain levels and superimposed on corresponding axial MRI slices (slice levels are 56 mm (top) and 42 mm (bottom) above the bi-commissural plane). This single subject was shown a visual fixation point and was asked to perform first horizontal self-spaced saccades. Blood flow evaluated by standard techniques using oxygen-15 was compared with a rest condition during which the subject fixated the visual target. Colour scale represents CBF increase in pixel counts normalised by whole brain counts. R, right; L, left. The subject was then asked to fixate the visual target and simulate mentally imagined saccades similar to the previously executed ones. Eye movements were measured by electro-oculography. This picture shows that in both cases the SMA and the frontal eye field were activated. The precision of the technique does not allow for a dissociation between several subparts of the SMA or FEF (from Lang, et al. 1994)

We even proposed some years ago that adaptive changes could also be obtained by mental effort and showed that this was true in the case of prism, adaptation (Melvill Jones and Berthoz 1985; Melvill Jones et al. 1984).

In summary all of the above considerations point to the necessity take into account the fact that the brain is 1) a predictive biological machine, 2) a simulator of action in order to predict the consequences of action by referring to past experience, and 3) probably using for these purposes inner loops in which action is simulated (and not represented) in extremely specialised circuits. In this perspective, "free will" is nothing other than the capacity to internally simulate action and make a decision, i.e., selectively remove inhibitions at many levels of the central nervous system and generate an executed or imagined action. We have to expect that this will be a hierarchy of neural decision processes allowing any intermediate process from quasi automatic very rapid sensori-motor decisions (like catch-avoid) to slow, memory based, social decisions.

References

Alexander GE, Delong MR, Strick PL (1986) Parallel organisation of functionally segregated circuits linking basal ganglia and cortex. Ann Rev Neurosci 9:357–381

Baker R, Berthoz A (1975) Is the prepositus hypoglossi nucleus the source of another vestibular ocular pathway? Brain Res 86:121–127

Berthoz A (ed) (1993a) Multisensory control of movement. Oxford University Press, Oxford

Berthoz A (1993b) Leçon inaugurale. Collège de France, Paris

Berthoz A, Grantyn A (1986) Neuronal mechanisms underlying eye-head coordination. In: Freund U, Buttner U, Cohen B, Noth J (eds) Progress in brain res earch. Elsevier, Amsterdam, pp 325–343

Berthoz A, Droulez J, Vidal PP, Yoshida K (1989) Neural correlates of horizontal vestibuloocular reflex cancellation during rapid eye movements in the cat. J Physiol London 419:717–751

Berthoz A, Mazoyer B, Petit L, Orssaud C, Raynaud L, Tzourio N (1992) Bilateral parietal involvement in the execution of a sequence memorized saccades in man. Soc Neurosci Abstr 18

Berthoz A, Pavard B, Young L (1975) Perception of linear horizontal self motion induced by peripheral vision (linear-vection). Exp Brain Res 23:471–489

Boussaoud D, Wise SP (1993) Primate frontal cortex: Neuronal activity following attentional versus intentional cues. Exp Brain Res 95:15–27

Boussaoud D, Barth TM, Wise SP (1993) Effects of gaze on apparent visual responses of frontal cortex neurons. Exp Brain Res 93:423–434

Brandt T, Dichgans J, Koening E (1973) Differential effects of central versus peripheral vision on egocentric and exocentric motion perception. Exp Brain Res 16:476–491

Büttner U, Henn V (1981) Circularvection: Psychophysics and single-unit recordings in the monkey. Ann NY Acad Sci 374:274–283

Curthoys IS, Markham CH, Furuya N (1984) Direct projection of pause neurons to nystagmus related excitatory burst neurons in the cat pontine reticular formation. Exp Neurol 83:414–422

Damasio AR (1994) Descartes' error. Emotion, reason and the human brain. Grosset/Putnam's, New York

Damasio AR, Tranel D, Damasio H (1991) Somatic markers and the guidance of behavior: Theory and preliminary testing. In: Levin HS, Eisenberg HM, Benton AL (eds). Frontal Lobe Function and Dysfunction. Oxford University Press, New York, pp 217–229

de Graaf B, Wertheim AH, Bles W, Kremers J (1990) Angular velocity, not temporal frequency, determines circular vection. Vision Res 30:637–646

Decety J, Michel F (1989) Comparative analysis of actual and mental movement times in two graphic tasks. Brain Cognition 11:87–97

Decety J, Perani D, Jeannerod M, Bettinardi V, Tadary B, Woods R, Mazziotta JC, Fazio F (1994) Mapping motor representations with PET. Nature 371:600–602

Deniau JM, Chevalier G (1981) Disinhibition as a basic process in the expression of striatal functions. The striatonigral influence on thalmo-cortical cells of the ventromedial thalamic nucleus. Brain Res 334:227–233

Dichgans J, Brandt T (1978) Visual-vestibular interactions: Effects on self-motion perception and postural control. In: Leibowitz H, Teuber HL (eds) Handbook of sensory physiology. Vol V. Springer, Berlin, New York, Heidelberg, pp 755–804

Droulez J, Berthoz A, Vidal PP (1985) Use and limits of visual vestibular interaction in the control of posture. Are there two modes of sensorimotor control? In: Igarashi M, Owen Black F (eds) Vestibular and visual control on posture and locomotor equilibrium. Karger, Basel, pp 14–21

Frith CD, Friston K, Liddle PF, Frackowiak RSJ (1991) Willed action and the prefrontal cortex in man: a study with PET. Proc Royal Soc London 244:2441–2246

Fuchs AF, Kaneko CRS, Scudder CA (1985) Brainstem control of saccadic eye movements. Ann Rev Neurosci 8:307–337

Funahashi S, Bruce C, Goldman-Rakic PS (1989) Mnemonic coding of visual space in the monkey's dorsolateral prefrontal cortex. J Neurophysiol 61:1–19

Funahashi S, Bruce CJ, Goldman-Rakic PS (1993a) Dorsolateral prefrontal lesions and oculomotor delayed-response performance: Evidence for mnemonic "scotomas." J Neurosci 13:1479–1497

Funahashi S, Chafee MV, Goldman-Rakic PS (1993b) Prefrontal neuronal activity in rhesus monkeys performing a delayed anti-saccade task. Nature 365:753–756

Gaymard B, Pierrot-Deseilligny C, Rivaud S (1990) Impairment of sequences of memory guided saccades after supplementary motor area lesions. Ann Neurol 28:622–626

Gaymard B, Rivaud S, Pierrot-Deseilligny C (1993) Role of the left and right supplementary motor areas in memory-guided saccade sequences. Ann Neurol 34:404–406

Gibson JJ (1966) The senses considered as perceptual systems. G. Allen and Unwin, London

Glimcher PW, Sparks DL (1992) Movement selection in advance of action in the superior colliculus. Nature 355:542–545

Goldman-Rakic P (1994) Cerebral cortical mechanisms in schizophrenia. Neuropsychopharmacoloty 10:22S–27S

Grantyn A, Berthoz A (1985) Burst activity identified tecto-reticulo-spinal neurons in the alert cat. Exp Brain Res 57:417–421

Grantyn A, Berthoz A (1987a) Reticulo-spinal neurons participating in the control of synergic eye and head movements during orienting in the cat. I. Reticulo-spinal neurons mediating eye head synergy during orienting in the cat. Exp Brain Res 66:339–354

Grantyn A, Berthoz A (1987b) The role of the tecto-reticulo-spinal-system in control of head movement. In: Peterson BW, Richmond FJ (eds) Control of head movement. Oxford University Press, Oxford, pp 224–244

Grantyn A, Grantyn R (1982) Axonal patterns and sites of termination of cat superior colliculus neurons projecting in the tecto-bulbo-spinal tract. Exp Brain Res 46:243–256

Grüsser OJ, Pause M, Schreiter U (1982) Neuronal responses in the parieto-insular vestibular cortex of alert Java monkeys (Macaca fascicularis). In: Roucoux A, Crommelinck M (eds) Physiological and pathological aspects of eye movements. Junk Publishers, The Hague, pp 251–270

Grüsser OJ, Pause M, Schreiter U (1990a) Localisation and responses of neurones in the parieto-insular vestibular cortex of awake monkeys (Macaca fascicularis). J Physiol 430:537–557

Grüsser OJ, Pause M, Schreiter U (1990b) Vestibular neurones in the parieto-insular cortex of monkeys (macaca fascicularis): visual and neck receptor responses. J Physiol 430:559–583

Guitton D, Buchtel HA, Douglas RM (1985) Frontal lobe lesions in man cause difficulties in supressing reflexive glance and in generating goal-directed saccades. Exp Brain Res 58:455–472

Hikosaka O, Wurtz RE (1983) Visual and oculomotor functions of the monkey substantia nigra pars reticulata: IV. Relation of substantia nigra and superior colliculus. J Neurophysiol 49:1285–1301

Hikosaka O, Sakamoto M, Usui S (1989a) Functional properties of monkey caudate neurons. I. Activities related to saccadic eye movements. J Neurophysiol 61(4):780–798

Hikosaka O, Sakamoto M, Usui S (1989b) Functional properties of monkey caudate neurons. II. Visual and auditory responses. J Neurophysiol 61(4):799:812

Hikosaka O, Sakamoto M, Usui S (1989c) Functional properties of monkey caudate neurons. III. Activities related to expectation of target and reward. J Neurophysiol 61(4):814–832

Hikosaka O, Sakamoto M, Miyashita N (1993) Effects of caudate nucleus stimulation on substantia nigra cell activity in monkey. Exp Brain Res 95:457–472

Joseph JP, Barone P (1987) Prefrontal unit activity during a delayed oculomotor task in the monkey. Exp Brain Res 67:460–468

Kaneko CRS, Evinger C, Fuchs AF (1981) Role of cat pontine burst neurons in generation of saccadic eye movements. J Neurophysiol 46:387–408

Keating EG (1991) Frontal eye field lesions impair predictive and visually-guided pursuit eye movements. Exp Brain Res 86:311–323

Lackner JR (1988) Some proprioceptive influences on the perceptual representation of body shape and orientation. Brain 111:281–297

Lackner JR, Levine MS (1979) Changes in apparent body orientation and sensory localization induced by vibration of postural muscles: vibratory myesthetic illusions. Aviation, Space Environ Med 50:346–354

Lacquaniti F (1989) Central representations of human limb movement as revealed by studies of drawing and handwriting. Neurosci 12:287–291

Lacquaniti F (1992) Automatic control of limb movement and posture. Curr Opin Neurobiol 2:807–814

Lang W, Petit L, Höllinger P, Pietrzyk U, Tzourio N, Mazoyer B, Berthoz A (1994) A positon emission tomography study of oculomotor imagery. Neuroreport 5:921–924

Llinas R (1974) La forme et la fonction des cellules nerveuses. La Recherche 43:232–241

Llinas R (1988) The intrinsic electrophysiological properties of mammalian neurons: insights into central nervous system function. Science 242:1654–1664

Mach E (1967) Grundlinien der Lehre von den Bewegungsempfindungen. Bonset, E.J. Amsterdam, pp 128

Magnin M, Jeannerod M, Putkonen PTS (1974) Vestibular and saccadic influences on dorsal and ventral nuclei of the lateral geniculate body. Exp Brain Res 21:1–18

Matsumoto N, Schwippert WW, Beneke TW, Ewert JP (1991) Forebrain-mediated control of visually guided prey-catching in toads: invstigation of striato-pretectal connections with intracellular recording/labeling methods. Behav Processes 25:27–40

Melvill Jones G, Berthoz A (1985) Mental control of the adaptative process. In: Melvill Jones G, Berthoz A (eds) Adaptative mechanisms in gaze control. Elsevier, Amsterdam, pp 203–208

Melvill Jones G, Berthoz A, Segal B (1984) Adaptative modification of the vestibulo-ocular reflex by mental effort in darkness. Exp Brain Res 56:149–153

Mistlin AJ, Perett DI (1990) Visual and somatosensory processing in the macaque temporal cortex: the role of "expectation". Exp Brain Res 82:437–450

Moschkovakis AB, Karabelas AB, and Highstein S (1988a) Structure function relationship in the primate superior colliculus. I. Morphological classification of efferent neurons. J Neurophysiol 60:232–262

Moschkovakis AB, Karabelas AB, Highstein S (1988b) Structure function relationship in the primate superior colliculus. II. Morphological identity of presaccadic neurons. J Neurophysiol 60:263–302

Park S, Holzman PS (1992) Schizophrenics show spatial working memory deficits. Arch Gen Psychiatr 975–982

Pierrot-Deseilligny C, Rivaud S, Gaymard B, Agid Y (1991) Cortical control of reflexive visually-guided saccades. Brain 114:1473–1485

Pierrot-Deseilligny C, Israël I, Berthoz A, Rivaud S, Gaymard B (1993) Role of the different frontal lobe areas in the control of the horizontal component of memory-guided saccades in man. Exp Brain Res 95:166–171

Posner MI, Walker JA, Friedrich FJ, Rafal RD (1984) Effects of parietal lobe injury on covert orienting of visual attention. J Neurosci 4:1863–1874

Premack D (1993) Prolegomenon to evolution of cognition. In: Poggio TA, Glaser DA (eds) Exploring brain functions: models in neuroscience. John Wiley and Sons Ltd, London, pp 269–290

Rizolatti G, Camarda R (1987) Neural circuits for spatial attention and unilateral neglect. In: Jeannerod M (ed) Neurophysiological and neuropsychological aspects of spatial neglect. Elsevier, Amsterdam, pp 289–313

Sauvan XM, Bonnet C (1993) Properties of curvilinear vection. Perception Psychophys 53:429–435

Yarbus AL (1967) Eye movements and vision. Plenum Press, New York

Yoshida K, McCrea RA, Berthoz A, Vidal PP (1982) Morphological and physiological characteristics of inhibitory burst neurons controlling horizontal rapid eye movements. J Neurophysiol 48:761–784

How the Basal Ganglia Make Decisions

G. S. Berns[1,2] and *T. J. Sejnowski*[1]

Abstract

The primate basal ganglia are a collection of subcortical structures that have long been considered part of the extrapyramidal motor system, the part of the motor system concerned with automatic aspects of movement. Despite a large amount of data regarding their anatomy and physiology, the role of the basal ganglia in both action planning and decision making remains enigmatic. Anatomical labeling studies have suggested that the striatum receives projections from the cerebral cortex that coarsely preserves topography, and that the basal ganglia maintain a segregation of information streams (Goldman-Rakic and Selemon 1986; Hoover and Strick 1993; Parent 1990). We suggest that the connectivity of the basal ganglia is ideally suited to selecting optimal actions for given cognitive and sensory states. We demonstrate how a computational network of pools of neurons connected in the arrangement found in the basal ganglia can perform what we term a "winner-lose-all" function. The winner-lose-all mechanism refers to the fact that the neurons of the output stage of the basal ganglia, the internal segment of the globus pallidus (GPi), are tonically active and are inhibited when corresponding striatal afferents fire. Thus the GPi neuron that is selected is actually inhibited because it loses rather than wins the competition. Diffuse excitatory projections from the subthalamic nucleus prevent all but the winning pallidal neuron pool from being inhibited. Because the thalamic targets of the GPi projection in turn feed back to the approximate cortical area of the originating afferent, this cortical-subcortical loop is ideally suited not only for the aforementioned action-selection, but also for the generation of sequences appropriate for given cortical states. We demonstrate how the circuitry of the basal ganglia can learn to select the best action for different cortical states and how the feedback representation of the action-selection leads to the generation of sequences of actions.

[1] Howard Hughes Medical Institute, Computational Neurobiology Laboratory, Salk Institute for Biological Studies, P.O. Box 85800, San Diego, CA 92186-5800, USA
[2] Present Address: Western Psychiatric Institute and Clinic, University of Pittsburgh Medical Center, 3811 O'Hara Street, Pittsburgh, PA 15213, USA

A.R. Damasio et al. (Eds.)
Neurobiology of Decision-Making
© Springer-Verlag Berlin Heidelberg 1996

Introduction

Decision-making occurs at several levels within the central nervous system. At the highest level, the individual consciously uses both past experience and future predictions to choose an action. At the lowest level, decisions are made that do not reach consciousness until after actions are performed, and the individual is unaware of the process leading up to the particular choice. We propose that the function of a large collection of subcortical structures, the basal ganglia, is to perform automatic decision-making. The basal ganglia have classically been considered primarily part of the extrapyramidal motor system, that is, the part of the motor system concerned with automatic movement, but a wealth of new data now supports an expanded role for the basal ganglia that includes an analagous function for cognitive processes.

The basal ganglia are a collection of subcortical structures whose anatomy and physiology have been characterized in great detail. The input stage, the striatum, receives a diverse input from virtually the entire neocortex. The striatum, which itself is subdivided into the caudate and putamen, preserves the topography of the glutamanergic, excitatory afferents from the cortex. Within the striatum, a high degree of modularity exists so that discrete compartments, termed matrisomes and striosomes, have interconnectivity within compartments, but not between them. This modularity will turn out to be crucial to the model we propose. The striatal projection neurons, which are GABAergic and inhibitory, project to the globus pallidus, which itself is comprised of an internal and external segment. Striosomes also project reciprocally to the substantia nigra, the brain's primary source of dopamine. The external segment of the globus pallidus (GPe) projects via GABAergic inhibitory neurons almost exclusively to the subthalamic nucleus (STN). The STN also receives an excitatory cortical input. The STN projects via diffuse excitatory neurons to the internal segment of the globus pallidus (GPi). Thus the GPi receives an inhibitory projection from the striatum and an excitatory projection from the STN. These opposing influences in the GPi will be central to our proposed mechanism of decision-making in the basal ganglia. The GPi, which is the output stage of the basal ganglia, projects via GABAergic neurons to the ventrolateral thalamus, which in turn projects back to the cortex, though not necessarily to the same neurons that formed the original loop.

The anatomy of the basal ganglia is unique in the brain in that 80% of the neurons are inhibitory, with γ-aminobutyric acid (GABA) as the main neurotransmitter. In particular, the striato-pallido-thalamic pathway is comprised of two GABAergic neurons in series, provoking the question of what the functional advantage of such an arrangement is over a monosynaptic excitatory pathway. Some degree of cortical topography is preserved throughout all the structures of the basal ganglia, with the exception of the substantia nigra (Parent 1990). This finding originally gave rise to the idea of multiple parallel streams of information circulating through the basal ganglia and back to the cortex without any significant integration (Alexander and Crutcher 1990; Alexander et al. 1986). However, the caudate and putamen receive afferents from diverse cortical areas, and then project in approximately a 1000:1 ratio to the globus pallidus (Wilson 1990). These two levels of convergence indicate either a substantial amount of integration or the multiplexed use of a structure by separate cortical areas. If integration is occurring, it most likely is computed in functionally discrete compartments. The existence of striosomes and matrisomes, in which virtually no neurons cross compartment boundaries, supports the idea of information integration, but only within defined regions corresponding to a particular action (Flaherty and Graybiel 1994; Graybiel 1990). The original hypothesis for parallel loops has now been modified, based on transneuronal retrograde tracing, to one of multiple segregated output channels (Hoover and Strick 1993). We took as our starting point the evidence for segregated channels corresponding to different possible actions, and show how the circuitry of the basal ganglia can effectively integrate several sensory and cognitive modalities to select one "best" action at any given moment.

Model

We modeled the basal ganglia as groups of simplified units interconnected according to the various divisions of the structure. Each unit corresponded to a locally distributed representation of some function, perhaps corresponding to a single matrisome in the striatum. These units were assumed to be functionally segregated and topographically related to the cortical targets that implemented the actions. The output stage of the basal ganglia, the GPi, is known to be almost wholly GABAergic and tonically active. Thus in our model the GPi tonically inhibits the target thalamic nuclei (VLm, VLpc/mc, VLo, CM). Because these nuclei also gate ascending information to their cortical targets (motor, supplementary motor, prefrontal cortices), it is reasonable that they should be tonically inhibited until the ascending information is required for action. Given that the GPi neurons must be tonically active in order for one information stream to be selected, one GPi unit must be turned off, thus allowing for disinhibition of the corresponding thalamic target. In connectionist terminology, this is thought of as a "winner-take-all" mechanism, but here it is more accurately termed a "winner-lose-all" because the selected GPi target turns off. Because the GPi unit must be inhibited, the afferent projections to the GPi, from the neostriatum, must themselves be inhibitory.

To implement the winner-lose-all mechanism, only one unit should be allowed to become inhibited. This was achieved by lateral excitation from the STN. As shown in Figure 1, the striatal, GABAergic neurons project in a parallel fashion to the GPi, but the striatal neurons also project in a convergent fashion to the GPe. The GPe, which is also tonically active, inhibits the STN. The first striatal neuron to reach firing threshold disinhibits its corresponding thalamic target (via the GPi), but it also disinhibits the STN (via the GPe). The firing of the STN excites a larger group of GPi neurons, thus preventing any other streams from being disinhibited. Because there was an extra delay associated with traversing the GPe/STN route, the so-called indirect pathway (Alexander and Crutcher 1990), any stream to be selected must inhibit the corresponding GPi target before the STN fires.

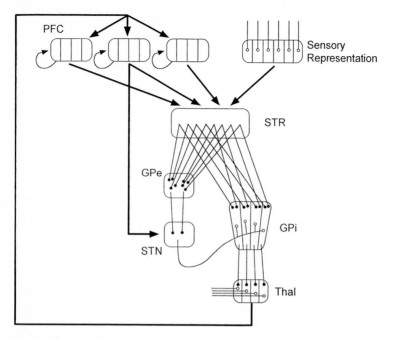

Fig. 1. Schematic diagram of the proposed winner-lose-all model of basal ganglia function. A multimodal sensory and cognitive map from the cortex projects in a convergent manner to the striatum. The prefrontal cortex (PFC) is represented as a site of working memory and contains copies of the thalamic output integrated over different time scales. The sensory representation roughly represents the parietal cortex and sends a processed representation of the environment to the striatum. The striatum (STR) sends two projections: a highly convergent one to the globus pallidus externus (GPe) and a moderately convergent one to the globus pallidus internus (GPi). The first pool of striatal neurons to reach firing threshold inhibits its target in the GPi. Inhibition of the GPi neuron leads to disinhibition of the corresponding thalamic neuron (Thal) and consequent gating of ascending information to the corresponding cortical motor neurons. Simultaneously, inhibition of the GPe neuron leads to disinhibition of the subthalamic (STN) neuron, which then diffusely excites the other GPi neurons. The diffuse excitation prevents all but the first action from being selected. The cortico-STN pathway acts as negative feedback to prevent ongoing activity within the loop, ensuring that selected actions are turned off

The STN receives a prominent excitatory projection from the cortex. We propose that the function of this pathway is to inhibit actions that have recently been selected. As shown in Figure 2, the STN receives both striatal and cortical projections from two segregated loops. In the context of each individual loop, the recurrent thalamo-cortico-STN path acts to inhibit preexisting activity (note that the loop has only one inhibitory neuron, and thus it acts as negative feedback). In the context of multiple loops, the STN also serves to inhibit competing actions as described above.

The prefrontal cortex (PFC) assumes a prominent role in our model. One of the PFC's functions is thought to be related to working memory (Fuster 1993). As illustrated in Figure 1, we modeled the PFC as representing multiple copies of the

Fig. 2. Diagram of two segregated cortical-subcortical loops. The STN diffusely excites the GPi units, which is necessary for the winner-lose-all, or action-selection function. It also acts as the focal point for negative feedback within each loop, preventing chaotic oscillatory activity which would lead to either tremor in a motor loop or persistent thoughts within a cognitive loop

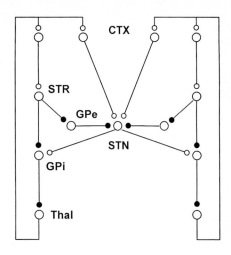

thalamus, in effect, multiple copies of the thalamic representation of the winning action. Each copy, however, represents an integration of activity on a different time scale. Thus the PFC contains several representations of previous winning actions, some representing recent activity and others representing the average activity over a longer time period. By virtue of the PFC-striatal projection, the decision-making function incorporates information about previously selected actions and thus can lead to the production of sequences of winning actions.

When a winner is selected, the action is assumed to be implemented through neurons in the cortical motor areas. The action results in some external event so that the model receives feedback regarding the appropriateness of the action performed. This feedback results in affective significance such that areas of the brain like the limbic cortex or the hypothalamus respond in an appropriate manner. Signals from these affective areas are presumed to reach several of the monoamine systems, which then release modulatory neurotransmitters. Montague et al. (1994) proposed a model of reinforcement learning in which the diffuse monoamine systems, especially the dopamine system, could modify synaptic strengths. They suggested that dopamine is released in response to deviations from learned predictions of future reward. Postulating that a diffuse neurotransmitter such as dopamine facilitates the change of synaptic strengths, they then demonstrated a plausible mechanism by which extrinsic rewards and penalties could be translated into the learning of specific behaviors. The primary source of dopamine, a neurotransmitter whose release is known to be closely linked to reward-driven behavior, is located in the ventral tegmental area (VTA), a structure also known to have intimate connections with the basal ganglia. Because of the close relationship with the action-selection model described above, we modeled the effect of dopamine as that of a neuromodulator that changes cortico-striatal synapse strength in close accordance with the Montague-Dayan-Sejnowski model (1994).

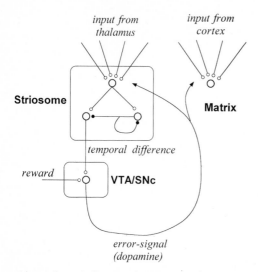

input from thalamus   *input from cortex*

Striosome   **Matrix**

temporal difference

reward   VTA/SNc

error-signal (dopamine)

Fig. 3. Schematic diagram of a striosome. The striosome computes a temporal difference of its inputs, which represent the predicted future reward associated with a particular action. The temporal difference estimates the correction to an earlier prediction, i.e., it approximates the error in the prior estimate. The striosome projects to the ventral tegmental area (VTA) and substantia nigra (SNc), where the temporal difference is combined with a representation of the actual reward received. The difference in these two inputs is diffusely projected back to the striatum via dopamine neurons to modify cortico-striatal synapses

The dopamine signal from the VTA represents a prediction error for all future rewards based on the current state of the brain. This pool of neurons receives a projection from the limbic system, which conveys the instantaneous reward or affective significance of an event. Another afferent comes from the patch component of the striatum. This striosome computes a modified temporal difference (Barto et al. 1990; Sutton 1988; Sutton and Barto 1990) of the expected reward associated with the action selected by the winner-lose-all mechanism (Fig. 3). There are two possibilities for conveying the information to the striatal patch about the selected action. One possibility is through the cortex; the other possibility, which we have used, relies upon the thalamo-striatal pathway, and in particular, the intralaminar nuclei.

Simulations

Each unit was modeled in terms of its firing rate. At each time step, a function was applied to each unit that took the sum of all its respective inputs, each of which represented the firing rate of an afferent unit multiplied by a factor proportional to the synaptic weight. For example,

$$y_i = g\left[\sum_j w_{ij} x_j\right] \tag{1}$$

where y_i is the output firing rate of cell i, w_{ij} is the synaptic strength from cell j to cell i, x_j is the firing rate of input cell j, and g is a sigmoidal function that has both upper and lower saturations so that a cell can neither have a negative firing rate nor exceed a maximum rate (see Fig. 4). Explicitly, the sigmoid function is given by:

$$g(x) = \frac{1}{1 + e^{-gain(x+bias)}} \tag{2}$$

where *gain* controls the slope of the inflection point and *bias* controls the shift. Table 1 provides the values for *gain* and *bias* for each of the units in the model.

The activity of each unit in the model was computed every millisecond, which corresponded to one time step. At each time step, activity was computed sequentially from the cortex to the thalamus. The input to the cortical units was

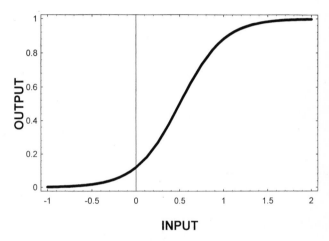

Fig. 4. General form of the input-output function of model units. The output represents firing rate. The input represents a sum of the afferent firing rates, but with each afferent weighted by the strength of its synapse to the unit. The sigmoidal function both prevents negative firing rates and allows for a maximum firing rate. The slope of the inflection point is determined by *gain* in Equation 2, and the location of the inflection point by *bias*. Here, **gain** = 4 and **bias** = −0.5

Table 1. Values for *gain* and *bias* in Equation 2 for the different synapses in the model

Synapse[a]	Gain	Bias
CTX → STN	+4	−0.5
STR → STN	+4	−0.5
STR → GPi	−4	−0.25
STN → GPi	+8	−0.25
GPi → Thal	−8	−0.5

[a] CTX, cortex; STR, striatum; STN, subthalamic neuron; GPi, internal segment of the globus pallidus; Thal, thalamus.

either an external input at the beginning of a run or the activity of the corresponding thalamic unit, delayed by 100 ms. When the cortico-striatal pathway is stimulated in vitro, an EPSP with irregular spiking is observed in the striatum, which is followed by another EPSP and spike 100 ms later (Wilson 1990), suggesting a 100 ms transit time for the whole loop. In order to model working memory in the PFC, the cortical units additionally had 20 ms time constants associated with their activity, allowing for short-term storage. The striatal activity was then computed based on the cortical activity. The GPi activity was computed by the sum of the striatal and STN inputs, with the appropriate signs, but the STN input to the GPi was delayed by 10 ms to account for the extra synapses in the indirect pathway. The output of the GPi was then used as the input to the thalamus.

Two types of model were examined. One model represented a single recurrent loop and the other represented two competing loops. In the single-loop model, we studied the role of the STN in stopping ongoing activity. In the two-loop model, we studied both the role of the STN in inhibiting competing actions and the sensitivity to firing thresholds in the striatum in relationship to other parameters of the model.

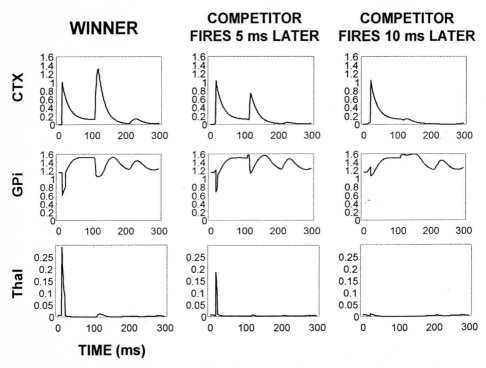

Fig. 5. Activity of the cortical (CTX), globus pallidus (GPi), and thalamic units (Thal) of two competing actions. The winning action (first column) is the first striatal unit to fire (at t = 0). There is a large thalamic discharge. A competing action is shown firing at both 5 and 10 ms after the first one. For longer delays, the transient decrease in GPi activity becomes progressively less, as does the corresponding thalamic disinhibition. This occurs because the winning action has already begun to diffusely excite the GPi units and thus prevents subsequent disinhibition of corresponding thalamic units

As an example of the winner-lose-all function, the efficacy of the STN in inhibiting competing actions is shown in Figure 5. The winning action corresponds to the striatal unit that fires first and results in the inhibition of the GPi unit, which in turn disinhibits the corresponding thalamic unit. A competing action in the two-loop model (Fig. 2) reaches firing threshold several milliseconds after the first one (Δt). When the second striatal unit fires, it has varying effects on the corresponding thalamic target because the first action has already started to diffusely excite the GPi units. When the second striatal unit fires at both 5 ms and 10 ms after the first, a markedly attenuated response is observed in its thalamic target.

In the context of a single recurrent pathway from cortex to striatum to globus pallidus to thalamus and back to cortex, the STN played a crucial role in preventing chaotic oscillations. As shown in Figure 6, the activity within a single loop without an STN unit was characterized by oscillations of activity at a frequency corresponding to the delay associated with the thalamo-cortex-striatum pathway (approximately 100 ms or 10 Hz). Without the STN unit, the presence of an initial stimulus led to oscillatory activity of chaotic amplitude, and in the absence of an initial stimulus, the loop activity was chaotic, but confined to a single basin of attraction (not shown). The addition of the STN unit effectively added negative feedback to the loop and prevented the ongoing oscillations after an initial stimulus. In effect, the STN acts as a brake following action selection.

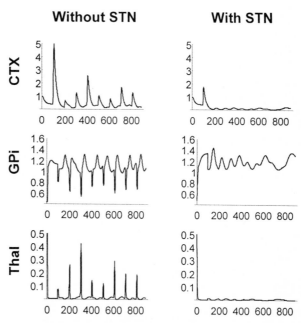

Fig. 6. Activity of cortical (CTX), globus pallidus (GPi), and thalamic units (Thal) with and without an STN unit in a single circuit. Without the STN, an initial stimulus to the cortical unit results in oscillations of chaotic amplitude throughout the circuit. With the STN, an initial cortical stimulus is subsequently inhibited by virtue of the GPi excitation. This prevents further periodic disinhibition of the thalamus (note that there is only one initial thalamic discharge)

Discussion

The proposal that the basal ganglia aid in decision-making was based largely on the observation that, given the existing anatomy of the basal ganglia, the connectivity of excitatory and inhibitory neurons is the simplest possible way to construct a winner-lose-all circuit. This proposed function is a fundamental prediction of our model that needs to be tested. The primary assumption for the winner-lose-all mechanism is the existence of streams of information that remain segregated from striatum to thalamus. We have formalized this segregation by representing each potential action by a separate unit, a so-called "grandmother cell;" however, this was chosen for computational efficiency. Each of the individual units in our model more realistically represents a pool of neurons devoted to a particular action, but the segregation requirement for pools of neurons remains.

Although there is good evidence for cortical topography being maintained throughout the basal ganglia (Alexander and Crutcher 1990; Alexander et al. 1986; Goldman-Rakic and Selemon 1986; Parent 1990), it is also known that the segregation is not complete. The massive convergence from striatum to globus pallidus (Wilson 1990) alone requires that inputs cannot remain completely segregated (Flaherty and Graybiel 1994; Hedreen and Delong 1991). However, our model is consistent with this convergence. We modeled the striatum as an input stage in which diverse areas of cortex map onto subsets of neuron pools. In this manner, diverse sensorimotor modalities are combined with higher representations of both context and timing information from the prefrontal areas. It is the functional mapping from striatum to globus pallidus and thalamus that remains segregated. In other words, the segregation may reflect the final cortical targets, not the afferents. Work with retrograde transneuronal transport of herpes simplex virus injected into the cortical motor areas suggests that the output stages of the basal ganglia are indeed organized into discrete channels that correspond to their targets (Hoover and Strick 1993).

To perform a winner-lose-all function, it was necessary to have a diffuse input to several neuron pools. We hypothesize that the "indirect" pathway (Alexander and Crutcher 1990) through the GPe and STN performs this function. Anatomically consistent with this hypothesis is the finding that the subthalamic inputs to the GPi are more diffuse than the striatal inputs (Hazrati and Parent 1992; Parent and Hazrati 1993). At the cellular level, the subthalamopallidal fibers appear as plexuses with varicosities, thus suggesting a diffuse excitatory function. A further requirement of our model is that subthalamic excitation overrides striatal inhibition. Hazrati and Parent (1992; 1993) reported that there is indeed a tendency for the subthalamic inputs to terminate proximally on the GPi neurons, whereas the striatal inputs terminate more distally in the dendritic tree. Such an arrangement would be consistent with excitation overriding inhibition.

The results of the model suggest that the efficacy of the winner-lose-all mechanism can be modulated by changing both the striatal resting membrane potential and the firing threshold. The resting membrane potential of both matrix and patch cells has been reported to be approximately $-70\,\mathrm{mV}$ (Kawaguchi et al. 1989);

The Will of the Brain: Cerebral Correlates of Willful Acts

D.H. Ingvar

Abstract

1. Current imaging techniques can depict physiological events in the brain which accompany sensory perception and motor activity, as well as speech. "Pure" mental events, unaccompanied by sensory input or motor/behavioral output, also induce different cerebral functional patterns related to inner representations of thoughts, ideas, visions, inner speech, etc.
2. Cognition, mental effort, and imagined volitional acts augment the activity in the frontal/prefrontal cerebral cortex. An augmentation in the cerebellum is also recorded. Temporally organized (serial) nerve cell activity takes place in these structures.
3. The prefrontal cortical activation accompanying volitional acts most likely corresponds to a willful mobilization of inner action programs which include representations of future events to be achieved by a goal-directed behavior.
4. Phylogenetically older parts of the cerebral cortex close to the midline (the cingulate gyrus) also participate in willful acts. Possibly they are involved in emotional/motivational ("value") aspects of volition.
5. Abnormal volition ("sick will") is encountered in organic dementia, Parkinson's disease, depression, and schizophrenia. Such disorders are characterized by inactivity, lack of ambitions, and a reduced motor and verbal output. Patients in these groups often show a decreased activity in prefrontal cortical regions.
6. Individuals with subfrontal and mesial frontal lesions may develop so-called psychopathic behavior with abnormalities of volition, lack of impulse control, boredom susceptibility, sensation-seeking behavior, and abnormal risk-taking.

Introduction

The basic function of the central nervous system is to translate sensory impulses into an adequate behavior. According to William James (1890) a prerequqisite for this translation is a "selection of stimuli and choice of response." To the

Department of Clinical Neurophysiology, University Hospital, 221 85 Lund, Sweden

A.R. Damasio et al. (Eds.)
Neurobiology of Decision-Making
© Springer-Verlag Berlin Heidelberg 1996

neurophysiologist there are, schematically, two main types of "choice of response:" One type is "automatic," reflexlike and directly stimulus-related. Such mainly non-conscious responses will not be considered here. The second type is coupled to a conscious attentional process, leading to a willed choice of a given response. This second alternative is combined with a suppression of other types of action.

The present review concerns regional cerebral functional (metabolic/circulatory) correlates to willful acts, as they can be measured by current brain imaging techniques. Indeed, there are also electrophysiological correlates of such acts in the brain, as shown clearly by Libet (1991), for example. Although his findings have several implications for the results reported below, they cannot be considered here.

The point of departure for the present review is an observation made nearly 20 years ago by Ingvar and Philipson (1977). Rhythmic, unilateral hand-clenching movements give rise to an activity peak in the contralateral hand area in the sensory-motor, *rolandic* region of the cerebral cortex. This finding confirmed the observations made by Olesen (1971). However, a willful conceptualization (inner representation) of the same rhythmic hand movement – without any motor activity – provided a different pattern, with mainly prefrontal cortical activation. This was the first direct evidence from brain imaging in conscious human beings that willful production of an internal representation of a movement (motor ideation) is accompanied by a frontal/prefrontal response located outside primary "executive" sensory-motor structures. Apparently, those parts of the cerebral cortex that program a given movement have a different location than the structures that control the execution of the actual movement.

In the present paper, emphasis is given to findings in normal subjects, but some observations in patients with various forms of "sick will" are also discussed.

Brain Imaging Techniques

The studies summarized below are based upon the principle of metabolic regulation of cerebral blood flow (Ingvar and Lassen 1975), i.e., that increased nerve cell activity in a circumscribed region of the brain is accompanied by a proportional increase of the metabolism, and of the regional cerebral blood flow (rCBF), in the same region. The opposite may also hold true, i.e., that diminished nerve cell activity lowers rCBF.

Originally, from the early 1960s and onwards, multiregional rCBF measurements were carried out following administration of an inert radioactive gas, 133 Xenon, dissolved in saline. Washout curves of 133 Xenon can be recorded externally over the brain, following either intra-arterial injection (Lassen and Ingvar 1961; Lassen et al. 1963, 1991; Ingvar and Lassen 1975) inhalation (Risberg 1980, 1986), or intravenous injection (Ryding 1986). The first studies were two-dimensional (2D), using multiple external detectors that depicted the distribution of function (rCBF) mainly in superficial cortical parts of the hemispheres. With these techniques the first "functional landscapes" in the human cerebral cortex were obtained. Later, three-dimensional (3D) single photon emission computer tomography (SPECT) techniques were developed for rCBF measurements in deeper parts of the brain (Stokely et al. 1980). Technical details of the 133 Xenon rCBF methods are described elsewhere (cf. Ingvar and Lassen 1975; Risberg 1986; Lassen et al. 1991; and Ryding et al., 1995).

The temporal and spatial resolution of the 2D rCBF measurements is relatively low, emphasizing activity changes in "outer," superficial parts of the hemispheres seen by external detectors. This may explain why 2D rCBF landscapes differ some-what from 3D SPECT or positron emission tomography (PET) studies. rCBF meas-urements with PET have a high spatial resolution, allowing subtle functional changes to be assigned to circumscribed regions in the cortex as well as in subcortical structures (Petersen et al. 1988; Posner et al. 1988; Frith et al. 1991; Raichle 1991; cf. Ingvar and Lassen 1975; Lassen et al. 1991). In spite of technical differences between earlier 2D and later 3D rCBF studies, most principal findings concerning willful acts appear to coincide.

For several years Jeannerod and his collaborators have been engaged in experimental and clinical studies of the neuropsychological basis of internal representations of movements. Their results have recently been reviewed by Jeannerod (1994). His extensive analysis, as well as the survey by Decety and Ingvar (1990), are referred to for neuropsychological concepts used in investigations of volition.

Consciousness and Will

In the present context, conscious awareness is considered a prerequisite for willful acts, which include active attentional mechanisms. Some current concepts about the neurophysiological basis of conscious awareness will therefore be reviewed.

The content of consciousness is, it must be assumed, temporally (serially, sequentially) organized. It encompasses information about serial events in the individual's past, present, and future. This information is willfully accessible more or less completely as an inner representation (overview) of one's life situation or "life time" (Ingvar 1983, 1985; cf. Fuster 1989; Edelman 1989; Searle 1992). Infor-mation about *past* events is retained as acquired memories, e.g., in the cortex of the temporal lobes and its deeper structures. Information about the *present* reaches the cortical sensory projection areas from the sensory organs. Information about the *future* is retained in frontal/prefrontal parts of the cerebral cortex as represen-tations of more or less complex action plans and behavioral programs (cf. Ingvar 1985; Goldman-Rakic 1988).

The tripartite information of one's past, present, and future can thus be localized – at least to some extent – in the brain (Ingvar 1985). During recall of memories of *past* events, an increased activity can be recorded in postcentral parts of the cerebral cortex and in certain subcortical structures (Roland and Friberg 1985; Goldman-Rakic 1988; Tulving et al. 1989). An increased sensory input – in the *present* – activates sensory projection areas of primary, secondary, or higher orders (Lassen et al. 1991). In addition, a general cortical activation dominating frontally can be recorded, especially if the sensory message requires cognitive effort and urgent handling (Risberg and Ingvar 1973; Risberg 1980, 1986). The imagination of *future* events activates specifically the frontal/prefrontal cortex (Ingvar and Philipson 1977; Risberg 1980, 1986), as shall be demonstrated. In this region there are neuronal networks that may retain activity for a certain time. They participate in "delayed responses" and in what is called "working memories" (Goldman-Rakic 1988, 1993; Fuster 1989). Apparently, they are involved in simple or complex neuronal programs for *future* actions. Such programs may form an integral part of inner representations.

Will as a Neurophysiological Concept

With the above background on conscious awareness, it should appear logical to presume that volition implies the mobilization of inner representations of *events in the future*. The goal which one "wills", i.e., wants to attain, is not present here and now, but only in the future. Inner goals, plans, concepts, expectations, and ambitions are coupled to motor and behavioral programs that are more or less clearly formulated to achieve the goal of the will.

Programs for willful acts also carry a "value," and emotional/motivational color of pleasure or displeasure. The goals of the willful act may be more or less desirable, more or less related to bodily or cognitive drives. The emotional color of an act of will is, it might be assumed, produced with the aid of the limbic system, in which basic and higher drives are generally believed to be controlled. However, emotional/drive aspects of will are not considered here, due to the lack of detailed knowledge about underlying cerebral mechanisms. In dealing with these issues we are approaching enigmatic problems related to will and the unconscious, a field that presently defies neurophysiological analysis (cf. Edelman 1989; Searle 1992).

Brain Images of Willful Acts

We have carried out 2D and 3D rCBF measurements in conscious human subjects performing willful movements and speech, as well as motor and speech ideation. Feedback effects to the brain from vocal and motor activity were avoided by using a paradigm comparing 1) the cortical landscape during an actual movement, during speaking aloud, during handwriting, etc., and 2) a second measurement during conceptualization of the same movement (motor ideation), during silent speech, or during imagining of handwriting, etc. The laboratory was kept silent during both studies, and in study 2 the subject was silent and motionless (no electromyographic activity). Simple, very brief controls of the inner willful representations were made, for example, by occasionally asking the subject how far he had come when counting silently or when imagining a series of writing movements

(Ingvar and Philipson 1977; Decety et al. 1988; Decety and Ingvar 1990; Friberg and Lassen 1991; Ryding 1989; Ryding et al. 1995).

The studies demonstrated that the performance of inner willful acts augmented the activity in frontal/prefrontal cortical regions, in which, as mentioned, action programs – for future use – are located. Bilateral rCBF measurements during silent speech further showed that the prefrontal activation was bilateral but asymmetrical (Ryding et al. 1995).

Prefrontal activation of the cerebral cortex during volitional acts has been confirmed and elaborated in PET studies of language paradigms or during motor and language performance in various combinations. Petersen et al. (1988; cf. Raichle 1991) demonstrated that a choice of semantically meaningful words resulted in circumscribed prefrontal activations. This finding was confirmed by Frith et al. (1991), who established different prefrontal rCBF patterns during willful choice of words as compared to willful finger movements. The specific content of the inner plan that guides the willful act thus puts an imprint upon the cortical landscape. Frith et al. (1991) further found that willful acts caused rCBF to decrease in certain cerebral regions. Such decreases may be coupled to suppression of alternative action plans that are not included in the chosen willful performance.

The PET studies cited above have shown that prefrontal mechanisms, connected to the dorso-lateral prefrontal cortex (DLPFC; Brodmann's area 46) on the left side, play a prominent role in volition. The importance of this area for delayed responses and so-called working memory has already been mentioned (Goldman-Rakic 1988, 1993).

We have also demonstrated in 3D SPECT measurements that the cerebellum is activated during willful ideation of motor acts or speech (Ryding et al. 1995; cf., Decety and Ingvar 1990). It thus appears possible that the cerebellum participates in the serial programming of motor acts and speech. Cerebellar mechanisms may form an integral part of the mental activity underlying the serial inner programming pertaining to volition.

Alterations of Consciousness and Volition

Conscious awareness is here considered a prerequisite for willful acts. Hence, alterations of consciousness to abnormally low or high levels may influence an individual's volitional capacity. This is in fact the case, as everyday experience tells us.

Low levels of awareness during drowsiness, exhaustion, lack of sleep, boredom, and for example the malaise caused by a common cold exemplify states in which it is difficult to perform willful acts. At even lower levels of brain activity, when one falls asleep, or during coma, the capacity to perform willful acts disappears completely.

At abnormally high levels of conscious awareness – during excitation, severe anxiety, pain with intense emotional stress, etc. – the realm of volition is also reduced. This appears to be due to the fact that anxiety and pain diminish one's ability to direct attention willfully.

States of the type mentioned, both "below" and "above" normal levels of conscious awareness, can be quantitatively defined in terms of a subnormal and supranormal, respectively, mean cerebral metabolism and blood flow. Thus an optimal level of brain activity might be established for an individual's volitional capacity. Such a general conclusion has in fact far-reaching implications, especially for individuals working in situations which demand constant willful decisions, such as in security jobs, military organizations, and the medical profession. Persons in charge of large organizations should also strive to retain an optimal volitional capacity by paying careful attention to their cerebral physiology.

A note on what is called "*collective will*" (Jung 1953) is justified here. This concept, frequently used in social psychology, has never been properly defined and related to pertinent physiological mechanisms. In view of the findings discussed above, one may surmise that a collective will entails a vision of future events and goals shared by groups of individuals, by a social class, etc. These groups might also share a collective experience of how to achieve their goals willfully. There would thus seem to be common factors – based upon brain physiology – between the will of an individual and that of groups of individuals.

The "Sick Will": Clinical Considerations

Disorders of will in patients with neurologic and psychiatric ailments are numerous. Some are encountered in patients with focal cerebral lesions, in which structural defects have impaired necessary input and output functions. In the present context such states, e.g., with paralysis, aphasia, etc., are of less interest since the main emphasis here is given to the highest organization of the neurophysiology of will.

A higher disorder of sick will is found in organic dementia and in depressive states, as well as in schizophrenia. A common denominater in these disorders is a general inactivity with inhibited motor output, reduced word fluency, lack of initiative and ambitions, and inability to organize willfully one's future. Advanced forms of organic dementia, especially of the frontal type (Brun and Englund 1981; Risberg 1986), as well as severe cases of depression and catatonic schizophrenia, may show a profound rigid immobility and mutism with a total lack of all signs of willed action.

Interestingly enough, imaging techniques have demonstrated that patients with 1) organic dementia (Ingvar and Gustafson 1970; Gustafson and Risberg 1974; Hagberg and Ingvar 1976; Risberg 1986), 2) advanced affective disorders of the depressive type (Baxter 1991), and 3) schizophrenia (Ingvar and Franzén 1974; Ingvar 1980, 1987; Weinberger et al. 1986; Warkentin et al. 1989) may show signs of reduced activity in the prefrontal cortex.

In our first study of schizophrenia (Ingvar and Franzén 1974) we noted that the prefrontal rCBF reduction correlated to symptoms of autism, inactivity, and "lack of will." In some of our studies mentioned above the low frontal rCBF has been located in the DLPFC area. It was also observed that this prefrontal region could not be activated by certain psychological tests, especially by the Wisconsin card sorting test, which requires frequent changes of serial willful decisions (Weinberger et al. 1986). When the symptoms of schizophrenia subsided due to medication, a normal activation of the frontal cortex could be recorded (Warkentin et al. 1989).

The prefrontal dysfunction in schizophrenia, and perhaps also in depression, may be coupled to a disorder of the basal ganglia, according to prevalent theories. Subcortical structures may indeed play a role in volition. Parkinson's disease, with its reduction of dopaminergic neurons in the basal ganglia, should be mentioned here. This disorder is characterized by a prominent inability to perform willful acts, to initiate such acts, and to produce a normal motricity in general. Traumatic frontal lobe lesions, which may, at least in the initial phase be accompanied by inactivity and reduced volition (Wirsén 1991), should also be mentioned.

The "sick will" pertaining to so-called psychopathic behavior may also deserve a remark. It includes a lack of impulse control, boredom susceptibility, and what has been termed sensation-seeking behavior. Individuals of this type, even if only with subtle "subclinical" symptoms, may indeed cause social and economic harm due to their lack of judgment, abnormal risk-taking etc. A basic defect in psychopathy might be defined as a lack of insight into the future consequences of one's willful acts in the present. It is well established that psychopathic behavior may occur in individuals who have suffered frontal, especially subfrontal, lesions (Blumer and Benson 1975; cf. Wirsén 1991).

Concluding Remarks

Brain imaging studies in normal subjects, and the clinical observations summarized above, provide strong support to the conclusion that normal volition requires intactness of prefrontal cortical mechanisms. They appear to be responsible for the inner representations, ideas, plans, expectations, visions, etc., which form an integral part of the phenomenon of will. Apparently, such representations are related to activity in neuronal networks that guide the production of, and produce the programs for, *future* willed motor acts, language expressions, cognitive activity, and goal-directed behavior. The brain is apparently capable of developing inner representations, visions, etc., of future events that are used in the execution of willful acts. Such acts include suppression or inhibition of alternative programs other than those chosen to achieve the given goal. The mechanisms of this inhibition are, however, incompletely understood. Frith et al. (1991) found a reduction of activity in certain brain regions during willful acts. Possibly this finding is related to inhibitory phenomena pertaining to the normal cerebral physiology of volition.

Finally, willful acts activate cingulate structures on the mesial side of the hemispheres (Frith et al. 1991). This finding suggests that brain mechanisms involved in the control of emotions, and in the "rating" of internal and external signals, participate in volition. Here we are approaching problems concerning drives, motivation and will. This important domain is difficult to discuss, in part due to our insufficient knowledge about the neurophysiology of the so-called subconscious.

References

Baxter LR, Guze BH, Schwartz JM, Phelps ME, Mazziotta JC, Szuba MP (1991) PET studies of cerebral function in major depression and related disorders. In: Lassen NA, Ingvar DH, Raichle ME, Friberg L (eds) Brain work and mental activity. Copenhagen, Munksgaard, 403–419

Blumer D, Benson DF (1975) Personality changes with frontal and temporal lesions. In: Blumer D, Benson DF (eds) Psychiatric aspects of neurological disease. New York, Grune & Stratton

Brun A, Englund E (1981) Regional pattern of degeneration in Alzheimer's disease: neuronal loss and histopathological grading. Histopathology 5:549–564

Decety J, Ingvar DH (1990) Brain structures participating in mental simulation of motor behaviour: A neuropsychological inter-pretation. Acta Psychol 73:13–34

Decety J, Philippon B, Ingvar DH (1988) rCBF landscapes during motor performance and motor ideation of a graphic gesture. Eur Arch Psychiat Neurol Sci 238:33–38

Edelman GM (1989) The remembered present. A biological theory of consciousness. New York, Basic Books

Friberg L, Lassen NA (1991) Language and the cerebral hemispheres: Impact of stimulous relevance and absence of lateralized activation response as revealed by rCBF studies. In: Lassen NA, Ingvar DH, Raichle ME, Friberg L (eds) Brain work and mental activity. Munksgaard, Copenhagen, 294–312

Frith CD, Friston K, Liddle PE, Frackowiak RSJ (1991) Willed action and the prefrontal cortex in man: a study with PET. Proc Roy Soc 244:241–246

Fuster JM(1989) The prefrontal cortex. Anatomy, physiology, and neuropsychology of the frontal lobes. 2nd ed. New York, Raven Press

Goldman-Rakic PS (1988) Topography of cognition. Parallel distributed networks in primate association cortex. Ann Rev Neurisci 14:137–156

Goldman-Rakic PS (1993) The issue of memory in the study of prefrontal function. In: Thierry A-M, Glowinski J, Goldman-Rakic PS, Christen Y (eds) Motor and cognitive functions of the prefrontal cortex. Berlin, Springer, 112–121

Gustafson L, Risberg J (1974) Regional cerebral blood flow related to psychiatric sumptoms in dementia with onset in the presenile period. Acta Psychiatr Scand 50:516–538

Hagberg B, Ingvar DH (1976) Cognitigve reduction in presenile dementia related to regional abnormalities of the cerebral blood flow. Brit J Psychiatr 128:209–222

Ingvar DH (1980) Abnormal distribution of cerebral activity in chronic schizophrenia. A neuropshysiological interpretation. In: Baxter D, Melneshuk B (eds) Perspectives in schizophrenia research. New York, Raven Press, 107–125

Ingvar DH (1983) Serial aspects of language and speech related to prefrontal cortical activity. A selective review. Human Neurobiol 2:177–190

Ingvar DH (1985) "Memory of the future:" an essay on the temporal organization of conscious awareness. Human Neurobiol 4:127–136

Ingvar DH (1987) Evidence for frontal/prefrontal cortical dysfunction in chronic schizophrenia. The phenomenon of "hypofrontality" reconsidered. In: Helmchen H, Henn FA (eds) Biological perspectives in schizophrenia. New York, Raven Press, 201–211

Ingvar DH, Franzén G (1974) Abnormalities of regional cerebral blood flow distribution in patients with chronic schizophrenia. Acta Psychiatr Scand 50:425–462

Ingvar DH, Gustafson L (1970) Regional cerebral blood flow in organic dementia with early onset. Acta Neurol Scand (Suppl 43) 46:42–73

Ingvar DH, Lassen NA (eds) (1975) Brain work Copenhagen, Munksgaard

Ingvar DH, Philipson L (1977) Distribution of cerebral blood flow in the dominant hemisphere during motor ideation and motor performance. Ann Neurol 2:230–237

James W (1980, repr. 1950) The principles of psychology. Dover, New York

Jeannerod M (1994) The representing brain. Neural correlates of motor intention and imagery. Behav Brain Sci in print 17:187–245

Jung CG (1953–1971) Collected Works. London, Routledge

Lassen NA, Ingvar DH (1961) The blood flow of the cerebral cortex determined by radioactive Krypton-85. Experientia 17:42–43

Lassen NA, Hoedt-Rasmussen K, Sörensen SC, Skinhöj E, Cronqvist S, Bodforss B, Ingvar DH (1963) Regional cerebral blood flow in man determined by Krypton-85. Neurology 13:719–727

Lassen NA, Ingvar DH, Raichle ME, Friberg L (eds) (1991) Brain work and mental activity. Copenhagen, Munksgaard

Libet B (1991) "Conscious vs. neural time." Nature 352:27

Olesen J (1971) Contralateral focal increase of cerebral blood flow in man during arm work. Brain 94:635–646

Petersen SE, Fox PT, Posner MI, Mintun MA, Raichle ME (1988) Positron emission tomographic studies of the cortical anatomy of single word processing. Nature 331:585–589

Posner MI, Petersen SE, Fox PT, Raichle ME (1988) Localization of cognitive functions in the human brain. Science 240:1627–1631

Raichle ME (1991) Studies of the processing of single words in normal human subjects with PET. In: Lassen NA, Ingvar DH, Raichle ME, Friberg L (eds) Brain work and mental activity. Copenhagen, Munksgaard, 315–323

Risberg J (1980) Regional cerebral blood flow measurements by 133-Xe inhalation: Methodology and applications in neuro-psychology and psychiatry. Brain Lang 9:9–34

Risberg J, Ingvar DH (1973) Patterns of activation in the grey matter of the dominant hemisphere during memorization and reasoning. Brain 96:737–756

Risberg J (1986) Regional cerebral blood flow. In: Hannay HJ (ed) Experimental techniques in human neuropsychology. Oxford, Oxford Univ. Press, 514–543

Roland PE, Friberg L (1985) Localization of cortical areas activated by thinking. J Neurophysiol 53:1219–1243

Ryding E (1986) Measurement of cerebral blood flow by intravenous administration of 133 Xenon. Theory technique and clinical applications. Thesis, University of Lund

Ryding E, Brådvik B, Ingvar DH (1995) Silent speech activates circumscribed speech centers selectively in the dominant hemsiphere. Brain Lang (in print)

Ryding E, Decety J, Sjöholm H, Stenberg G, Ingvar DH (1992) Motor imagery activates the cerebellum regionally. A SPECT rCBF study with 99 m Tc-HMPAO. Cog Brain Res 1:1–6

Searle JR (1992) The rediscovery of the mind. Cambridge, Mass., MIT Press

Stokeley EM, Sveinsdottir E, Lassen NA, Rommer P (1980) A single photodynamic computer-assisted tomograph (DCAT) for imaging brain function in multiple cross-sections. J Comp Assist Tomogr 4:142–148

Tulving E, Risberg J, Ingvar DH (1989) Quoted from E. Tulving. Remembering and knowing the past. American Scientist, July–Aug

Warkentin S, Nilsson A, Risberg J, Carlson S (1989) Absence of frontal lobe activation in schizophrenia. J Cereb Blood Flow Metab (Suppl 1) 9:5354

Weinberger DR, Berman KF, Zec RF (1986) Physiological dysfunction of the dorsolateral prefrontal cortex in schizophrenia. 1. Regional cerebral blood flow (rCBF) evidence. Arch Gen Psychiat 43:114–125

Wirsén A (1991) Chronic effects of traumatic frontal lesions. Clinical, neurophysiological and neuropsychological aspects. Thesis, University of Lund

Neuronal Models of Cognitive Functions Associated with the Prefrontal Cortex

J.-P. Changeux[1] and *S. Dehaene*[2]

Summary

Understanding the neural bases of cognition has become a scientifically tractable problem, and neurally plausible models are proposed to establish a causal link between biological structure and cognitive function. To this end, levels of organization have to be defined within the functional architecture of neuronal systems. Transitions from any one of these interacting levels to the next are viewed in an evolutionary perspective. They are assumed to involve:

1. the production of multiple transient variations and
2. the selection of some of them by higher levels via the interaction with the outside world.

The time scale of these "evolutions" is expected to differ from one level to the other. In the course of development and in the adult, this internal evolution is epigenetic and does not require alteration of the structure of the genome. A selective stabilization (and elimination) of synaptic connections by spontaneous and/or evoked activity in developing neuronal networks is postulated to contribute to the shaping of the adult connectivity within an envelope of genetically encoded forms. At a higher level, models of mental representations, as states of activity of defined populations of neurons, are suggested and their storage is viewed as a process of selection among variable and transient "pre-representations" via a selective reward mechanism. Models are presented which can perform the delayed response task or the Wisconsin card sorting test and cognitive functions such as short-term memory, reasoning and handling of temporal sequences. Implementations of these mechanisms at the cellular and molecular levels are proposed. Finally, speculations are offered about plausible neuronal models and selectionist implementations of intentions.

Introduction

In biology, as in physics, the theoretical approach precedes experiment. Knowledge progresses by "conjecture and refutation" (Popper 1963), by the construction

[1] Institut Pasteur, 25, rue du docteur Roux, 75015 Paris, France
[2] Lab. des Neurosciences Cognitives, 54, Bld. Raspail, 75006 Paris, France

A.R. Damasio et al. (Eds.)
Neurobiology of Decision-Making
© Springer-Verlag Berlin Heidelberg 1996

of models followed by submitting them to the experimental test. Any model is a "representation" of a natural object or process described in a coherent, non-contradictory and minimal form, if possible mathematical. To be useful, the way in which it is formulated must allow comparison with outside reality. However, it cannot be expected that it will offer an exhaustive description of the latter. It may eventually be adequate, but will always remain limited.

Claude Bernard introduced a major distinction into life sciences by comparing anatomy (stable morphological organizations or "structures") with physiology (the dynamic processes by which an organism acts on the outside world or on itself). From there, the purpose of life sciences has become more precisely the determination of causal relationships between structure and function. This determination of relationships acquires a new dimension in the case of higher brain functions, where what is revealed of the mental state is still very often deliberately dissociated from subjacent neural organizations. Our purpose is completely opposed to any approach of this type since, in contrast, it concerns the creation of "a bridge" between neural sciences and mental sciences by developing neuronal models of cognitive functions.

Under these conditions, models of this type must be plausible at the neurobiological level and not merely be "artificial", which would exclude from the start any comparison with neuronal reality. To be adequate, it is also necessary that the strucure-function relationship should provide correspondence between theoretical and experimentally observable variables in a pertinent manner and particularly at the level of organization involved (Changeux and Dehaene 1989).

As the physician P. Anderson wrote in 1972 "the ability to reduce everything to simple fundamental laws does not imply an ability to start from these laws and reconstruct the universe." The organization of living beings must be considered within the context of the evolution of species, and this evolution shows a consistent increase in complexity during palaeontological history. A first theoretical and essentially qualitative approach is to break down these complex organizations into hierarchical levels of organization whereby their appearance during evolution coincides with the appearance of new functions. For F. Jacob (1970), "living beings are therefore constructed by means of a series of packages. They are fitted together according to a hierarchy of discontinuous units or integrons." Nerve cells are composed of molecules, but are assembled together into networks by dendrites and axons. The extension of this paradigm to clusters of neurons leads to differentiation of levels of organization within the brain itself. This must not be confused with the "levels" which Marr (1982) distinguishes in "Vision":

1. the "hardware" or neural machine;
2. the representation and algorithm and,
3. the computational theory.

In this case it concerns levels of understanding according to a scheme which perpetuates the cleavage between structure and function. This distinction may be useful for defining experimental pathways of approach or even for describing the system and its functional properties. However, it by no means takes any account of the levels of organization or of integration properly speaking and which may each highlight, at least in part, a description according to the terms of Marr.

Several models of the cleavage of functional brain organization into distinct "levels of integration" may therefore be proposed. Initially, the following levels were separated:

1. the level of elementary circuits and simple reflexes or fixed schemes of action (Kant's "sensitivity"?);
2. that of "groups of neurons" and of "symbolic representation" (Kant's "intendment"?);
3. that of complex assemblies of neuronal groups that we may refer to as "reason" (Kant) or "knowledge" (Newell) level (Newell 1982; Dehaene and Changeux 1989). However, we must expect even finer hierarchical cleavages.

The transition from one level of organization to the next is considered within the general conceptual context, which in this laboratory (Changeux et al. 1973; Changeux 1983) has always been that of an evolutionary epistemology (Popper 1966; Campbell 1974) inspired from Darwin's ideas (Darwin 1859; Poincare 1913) based upon:

1. a "blind" "generator of diversity" which introduces "variations" into the functional organization at the level being considered;
2. a mechanism of conservation and/or of propagation of the selected variation.

Within the context of the Darwinian scheme of evolution of species, variation occurs at the genome level (mutations, chromosome rearrangements, etc.), and the conservation of variations is performed by conservative replication of DNA and by propagation via sexual reproduction.

The application of this paradigm to the "internal" levels of organization of the brain does not postulate covalent variation of the genome but, in contrast, "epigenetic" variations of connectivity during development (time scale: years, minutes) or states of activity of neuronal clusters at level of symbolic representation or architectures of reason (time scale: 0.1 second, minute). The proposed models (Dehaene and Changeux 1989, 1991) relate to the general problem of transition from the "symbolic" level to the "reason" level (Changeux and Dehaene 1989), dealt with in the particular example of the prefrontal cortex.

Functional Organization of the Prefrontal Cortex

The prefrontal cortex is the region of the neocortex in which the surface area has increased relatively most during the course of mammalian evolution; it increases from 3.5% in the cat to 17% in the chimpanzee and, finally, 29% in humans (see Fuster 1989). Its histological organization is not uniform. In the 19th century, Brodmann subdivided the prefrontal cortex into several distinct territories, essentially on an anatomical basis. However, the latter mainly shows the six layers characteristic for the entire associative cortex, with a well-differentiated granular layer IV. The connectivity of the hundreds of millions of neurons which compose it (900 millions according to some estimates) is one of extreme richness; this is most often established in a reciprocal or "re-entrant" manner according to Edelman's (1978) term between the intrinsic neurons which compose it, but also with the neurons of many regions of the encephalon. The frontal cortex exchanges connections with regions of the cortex which are hierarchically inferior to it, parieto-temporal associative areas, then primary sensory areas and motor areas. Of all the cortex, it is the domain which is most densely connected with the limbic system, which, as is known, participates in emotional responses. It is also linked to the thalamus as well as to the basal ganglia, which are involved in the control of movement. Finally, several nuclei of the reticular formation and of other regions (containing neurotransmitters such as dopamine, noradrenaline, acetylcholine etc.) send highly divergent axons towards the frontal cortex where they control activity in a "global" manner. Examination of the connectivity of the frontal cortex allows at least three levels of hierarchical organizations to be defined, 'nested" (Campbell 1974) one within the other. Very schematically, the prefrontal cortex is surrounded by an inferior level which corresponds to the areas of association, and by a more global level represented by the reticulo-frontal loops.

As Harlow noted in 1868, lesions of the frontal lobe in humans are accompanied by emotional disorders (hyperemotivity, character instability; Nauta 1971) as well as profound "cognitive" disorders which are expressed both by excessive obstinacy (perseverance in error) and then abnormal tendency to distraction, with a general decrease in critical activity. For Diamond (1988) the frontal cortex ensures "the correlation of information with space or time" and "inhibits dominant action tendencies." It constructs and updates "representations of the environment" (Goldman-Rakic 1987) which allow the subject to "plan and elaborate anticipations" (Teuber 1964, 1972) of actions on the surrounding world. For Shallice (1982) it constitutes a system of "supervisory attentive system", hierarchically superior to the "routine" "contention scheduling" system. It ensures the construction of plans in non-routine situations and selects schemes appropriate to those situations, all the while recording and taking into account errors likely to intervene in the realization of the plan. The prefrontal cortex produces "mental syntheses" (Bianchi) and is the site of "intentional behaviour" (Pavlov). It is also involved in making decisions and forming plans in relation to social behavior (Damasio et al. 1991 and this volume).

It may be suggested that it corresponds to the "knowledge level" which theoreticians of artificial intelligence (Newell 1982) locate above the "symbolic" level and which may be the homologue of the "reason" level. Under these conditions, the prefrontal cortex would participate in the neural architectures of reason (Changeux 1988).

Functional Analysis of the Prefrontal Cortex by Various Tasks with Delayed Responses

In 1914, Hunter developed a behavioral test called the "delayed response task" which has since been very widely used with laboratory animals and even with children for the experimental analysis of prefrontal functions (Diamond 1988; Piaget 1954; Fuster 1984; for review see Dehaene and Changeux 1989). The experimental design is as follows. A stimulus or cue object is initially presented to the subject at a precise point in a scene, then a screen falls and covers the scene from the subject's sight for a variable duration; two objects are then presented at two different sites and the subject must choose one of the two. The rule defining the correct choice varies with the type of task involved. In the delayed response (DR) task in its strict sense, and in task AB̄ (A not-B; Piaget 1954), the rule is to choose the object which is located in the position occupied by the cue before the interval. In the DR task, the position of the cue is changed at random from one test to another, whereas in task AB̄ its position is changed only after the child has been successful in accomplishing the task. In the so-called "delayed matching-to-sample" task (DMS), the subject must choose an object identical to the cue irrespective of its position. Finally, a third task, called delayed alternation (DA), may be considered as part of this group of tasks. After having successfully performed a task at a given position, the subject must choose the alternative position in the following response. In all of these protocols, the subject learns the task during a training phase in which he receives the reward for each successful test (fruit juice in the monkey, playing with a toy in the case of children, etc.).

In all cases these are sensory-motor tasks which involve short-term memory of the subject and require selective attention. During the task, the subject makes a decision by comparing a test object with a memorized representation of the cue object. Finally, during training the subject performs an induction process in time and space by discovering the abstract rule (pertinent choice of feature) which governs the reinforcement.

In young children, systematic success in the AB̄ test develops around the age of 7.5 months and performances improve up to 12 months. The young macaque monkey masters these two tests between 1.5 and 4 months, and ablation of the frontal cortex at birth interferes with mastery of the test. In the absence of the delay, an immature subject or injured adult passes the test but, if the delay exceeds 1–2 seconds, performance deteriorates and essentially becomes random (for review see Diamond 1988).

The delayed response task reveals early "cognitive" functions which are nevertheless of a high order and linked to the integrity of the prefrontal cortex.

Electrophysiological Recordings During the Execution of a Delayed Response Task

To our knowledge, only a few rare electrophysiological data exist on the acquisition of mastery of the delayed response task (Kubota and Komatsu 1985). The principal data available are recordings of individual neurons in the monkey (macaque) during the performance of the DR test after training (for review see Fuster 1989; Funahashi et al. 1993; Watanabe 1986a). Neurons of a first type come into action when the cue is presented (Fuster 1973; Niki 1974, 1975). Their activity represents either an invariant early response appropriate to the task, which relates to the focussing of attention on the cue, or a response to the test itself, which distinguishes one cue from another, or finally, in some cases, both. Neurons of a second type, most often excitatory, change their activity in relation to the execution of the task; in general, their activity varies with the direction of movement of the hand which is required in the execution of the task (Kubota and Niki 1971; Watanabe 1986b). Their most remarkable feature is that their activity may anticipate the motor response by several seconds. Finally, the neurons of a third type are permanently active during the delay period, sometimes for a minute or more. Cells of this type are also encountered in the medio-dorsal thalamus and also in the temporal cortex, but to a much more limited degree. Neurons of this type are only observed in animals which have undergone training (it therefore does not concern a delayed sensory discharge). In addition, their activity is related to the state of alertness of the animal. Finally, there is a correlation between the activity of the cells during the delay period and the success of performance (distraction of the animal by an auditory stimulus during the delay period interferes both with the delay period activity and with success in the test). These neurons therefore establish a "temporal contingency" between presentation of the cue and motor performance. Their activity is not uniform. The discharge of a fraction of these cells tends to diminish during the delay period; these are short-term memory cells which participate in retention of the "representation" of the stimulus. The frequency of discharge of another fraction of neurons increases with time; they correspond to motor anticipations which prepare for movement. Coordination of the activity of these two categories of neurons ensures integration between short-term memory and preparation for motor action. Some cells which become temporarily active during the delay periods may participate in this coordination (Batner et al. 1981). At the end of the test, some prefrontal cells become active when the animal receives the reward and drinks the few drops of fruit juice received for a correct response. In contrast, other cells become active when the reward is expected but is not received (Rosenkilde et al. 1981).

These different types of cells are found throughout the prefrontal cortex; some are present in greater abundance in certain areas. The "reward" cells are present in the orbital regions, richly connected to the limbic system. The cells which are activated (or inhibited) during the delay period are mainly found in the region of the main sulcus of the dorso-lateral prefrontal cortex (Fuster 1989; Wilson et al. 1993).

A Model of the Formal Neuron Network Accomplishing the Delayed Response Test

The objective of this modeling (Dehaene and Changeux 1989) is to construct a minimal and biologically plausible neuronal network which successfully passes the delayed-response task. Such a network must allow identification of the critical elements which are necessary for success in the task, and prediction of new properties subject to experimental validation.

The Formal Organism and Its Environment

The formal neuronal network is contained in a "formal organism" which interacts with a very restricted environment. This environment is a priori limited initially to the objects serving as a cue, then to some pertinent features of the latter which are likely to be taken into account by the formal organism: position (dimension 1), with two possibilities, right or left; color (dimension 2) with three possible hues; and finally no more than two objects may be presented to the formal organism at any given moment.

Each task is composed of successive tests and each test comprises four stages: presentation of an object, interval in the absence of the cue object, presentation of two objects, choice of object with reward or punishment, and an interval between two tests.

In tests of type 1 (analogues of DR or $A\bar{B}$), the correct object is the one having a position (dimension 1) coinciding with that of the cue; in those of type 2 (analogues of DMS), the correct choice is that of color of the cue (dimension 2).

The reward (or punishment) signal is applied from outside (by a master who decides his mark) or, under more natural conditions, as a result of the sensory qualities (taste, nutritional value, etc.) which are intrinsic to the object and recognized by the organism as favorable (or unfavorable) to survival (as a result of its past evolution). The reinforcement parameter covers an interval $[-1, +1]$ where 0 is neutral, $+1$ is maximum reward and -1 is maximum punishment.

Elementary Components of the Network

The network is composed of "formal neurons" of the McCulloch and Pitts type (1943) (see Amit 1989 for discussion), linked together by synaptic contacts of either the excitation or the inhibitory type. Each neuron is able to exist in two states, active (discharge) or inactive (rest). However, the states of activity of individual neurons (or synapses) are not explicitly modelled.

The basic unit of the network is a "cluster of synergic neurons", the state of activity of which is assumed to code for an elementary "neural representation." This latter is analogous to Mountcastle's elementary module or "column" (Mountcastle 1978) or to Edelman's "group" of neurons (1978). It is defined and formalized here (Dehaene et al. 1987) as one hundred (or several hundred) neurons densely interconnected by excitatory synapses and, because of this, likely to exist in two self-sustained states of activity with either a high or a low frequency of discharge.

The neuron clusters are linked together by "axon bundles" of two types. The static bundles, not modulated by the activity of the network, propagate either lateral inhibition between clusters or the output of calculations performed by groups of clusters (or assemblies). The efficacy of the modulated bundles, for example between A and B, is regulated (to a maximum value) by the activity of a third neuronal cluster, for example C, called a modulator. The maximum efficacy value reached is itself variable and regulated by training (see below). Regulation of synaptic efficacy between A and B is undertaken in a "heterosynaptic" manner by

Environment   of   formal   organism

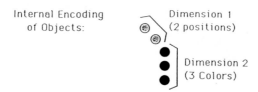

Internal Encoding
of Objects:

Dimension 1
(2 positions)

Dimension 2
(3 Colors)

Components   of   the   neural   network

formal   neurons

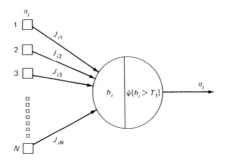

clusters   of   synergic   neurons

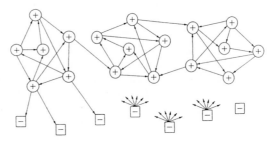

bundles   of   connections   &   synaptic   triads

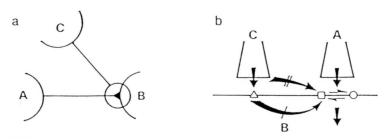

Fig. 1. Synaptic triad. Signals from synapse C-B modulate the efficacy of the neighboring A-B synapse. b is an enlarged view of a (taken from Dehaene et al. 1987)

C according to the "synaptic triad" scheme (Fig. 1) (Dehaene et al. 1987) where the signal produced by synaptic terminal C acting on neuron B regulates, by an extra- or intracellular signal, the allosteric transitions (Heidmann and Changeux 1982; Changeux and Heidmann 1987) of the postsynaptic receptor of synapse A → B. All the synaptic triads between neurons belonging to clusters of neurons A, B or C constitute a "modulated bundle."

Architecture of the Network

A major feature of the architecture of the network is its differentiation into two hierarchical levels of organization (Fig. 2). Level 1 (or execution level) includes two layers of neuron clusters, respectively "input" and "output." Each of the characteristic features of a given object is analyzed and coded by a particular cluster of input neurons. The output clusters are connected in an isomorphic manner with the input clusters, and the activity of the output clusters governs the orientation of the organism towards a defined object possessing a particular feature. Level 2 (or regulation level) includes a layer of "memory clusters" and a layer of "rule-coding clusters," and controls the processing of an object according to a defined rule. The memory clusters, which are self-excitatory and mutually inhibitory, project isomorphically and modulate the input-output connections. Each cluster of rule-coding neurons codes not for a particular feature of the object but for one

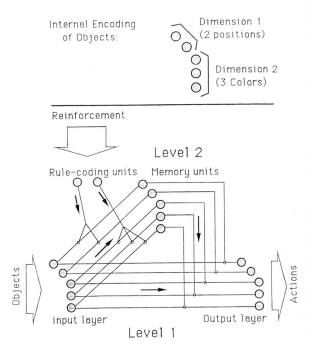

Fig. 2. Model of the role of the frontal cortex in learning and execution of delayed response tasks (taken from Dehaene and Changeux 1989)

dimension which groups together several features of the object (in the very restricted case of the proposed model, there are only two). The clusters of rule-coding neurons project onto bundles which link input clusters with memory clusters and regulate their efficacy. By analogy with the primate neocortex, level 1 would correspond to a visuo-motor loop which includes secondary visual areas and the motor (or pre-motor) cortex, and level 2 would be identified with the prefrontal cortex.

Learning a Behavioral Rule

The organism learns a defined behavioral rule by interpreting a reinforcement signal which governs both modifications of synaptic efficacy and random variations in spontaneous activity of clusters of rule-coding neurons.

The reinforcement (or reward) triggered "by return" as a result of the action of the organism on the environment during the learning process is "internalized" in the form of a parameter R which represents satisfaction (from 0 to + 1) or dissatisfaction (from 0 to − 1) of the organism. A first effect of R is to modulate the maximal efficacy of a synaptic triad according to Hebb's law. When R is positive and the postsynaptic neuron B (Fig. 1) is active at the same time, maximal efficacy increases; it decreases when the postsynaptic neuron is inactive. When R is negative, the rule is reversed.

Application of this rule is based on the allosteric properties of the postsynaptic receptor of synapse A → B. It is known that the nicotinic receptor for acetylcholine can exist in at least two desensitized states for which the ionic channel is closed (Changeux and Heidmann 1987). States I, of rapid access from the resting state, would be involved in the functioning of the synaptic triad. The fraction of receptors in state D, of slower access, would determine the maximum amplitude of variation in synaptic efficacy and is stabilized by the co-occurrence of two signals:

1. a postsynaptic signal (for example the intracellular concentration of Ca^{++}) which indicates recent activation of the cell, and
2. a diffuse extracellular signal (for example, the catecholamines of divergent reticulo-frontal pathways) which is propagated throughout all the synapses of the network for instance by "volume transmission" in the extracellular spaces (Fuxe and Agnati 1991; see Dehaene and Changeux 1991; Williams and Goldman-Rakic 1995).

A second effect of R is to modify the activity of clusters of rule-coding neurons. When the organism is dissatisfied, R becomes negative, there is destabilization of all the rule-coding clusters, and spontaneous activity then varies from one cluster to another.

Learning takes place by selecting a defined cluster of rule-coding neurons according to its actual state of activity. The layer of rule-coding clusters serves, in some way, as a Darwinian "generator of diversity" and its evolution in time is under the control of the reinforcement signal.

Functional Properties of the Model

Simulation of the behavior of a network comprising only level 1 shows that the organism which possesses it is able to learn as a result of the action of the reinforcement loop on the triads of the input-output "execution" network. In an $A\bar{B}$ test, it ceases to orient at random. There is acquisition of a systematic orientation towards position A for which it was trained when A and B were presented simultaneously. However, like all infants or monkeys before the development of efficient frontal connections, there will be systematic error when the position of the cue is changed from A to B. The organism which possesses only level 1 thus fails in the DR and DMS tasks. In contrast, it succeeds in all these tasks when it possesses levels 1 and 2.

The rule-coding neurons play a decisive role in the behavior of the organism. Their activity commands the memorization of a particular feature of the cue by modulating the efficacy of the connections between input clusters and memory clusters. If the rule-coding neurons which code for color are active, only the particular color of the cue will be memorized, but not its position. The neurons of the memory group themselves will govern the orientation of the organism towards the object possessing the memorized feature. In other words, the organism selects the object which possesses the characteristic feature of the cue to the extent that the rule-coding neurons which code for the particular category (position, color) to which this feature belongs are active.

The activity of the rule-coding neurons definitively "channels" the rule of behavior of the organism towards the choice. Learning therefore consists of a search among the various states of activity of rule-coding clusters to find the particular state which leads to the satisfaction of the organism. During learning, by successive "anticipations" based on the spontaneous variable and "blind" activity of rule-coding neuron clusters, the organism tests various features of the environment and selects the particular category of features of the object for which the "reward" is systematically positive.

The model allows simulation of the activity of defined neuron clusters during or after learning. In particular, neurons of the memory clusters display an activity which resembles that of neurons which are active during the delay period (see previous chapter) and the activity of which anticipates the behavior of the monkey during the choice when it is successful (but also when it fails; Fig. 3) (see Funahasi et al. 1993).

Simulation of the behavior of the formal organism shows that, with level 1 only, its behavior is analogous to the performances of infants aged from 7.5 to 9 months, of monkeys of 1.5 to 2.5 months or of monkeys with prefrontal lesions 17 (Fig. 4).

With level 2, the performances of the formal organism become practically identical to those of a child aged 12 months or of a rhesus monkey aged 4 months with respect to the learning of task $A\bar{B}$ or DMS. In addition, the organism is capable of passing from one task to another without difficulty.

Despite these successes, the formal organism modelled in this way presents three groups of limitations:

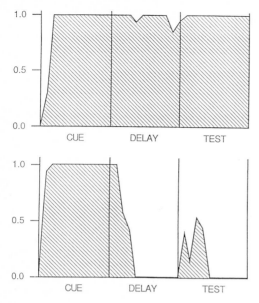

Fig. 3. Simulation of the activity of a memory neurons cluster during the delay. Top, the group remains active during the delay; performance in the next test is correct. Bottom, the group is inactivated due to internal noise; the organism now fails the test (taken from Dehaene and Changeux 1989). Similar data have been recorded in vivo with rhesus monkeys performing a delayed anti-saccade task (Funahashi et al. 1993)

1. the sensory-motor tasks are highly reduced in the number of sensory categories or features and types of motor behavior;
2. the architecture is extremely simple: the number of formal neurons is six-seven orders of magnitude lower than that of the neurons of the prefrontal cortex in humans: and
3. the range of available rules is very small in size.

With the purpose of extending this research to more complex functions and to richer networks, a modeling of the Wisconsin card sorting test was investigated (Dehaene and Changeux 1991).

The Wisconsin Card Sorting Test

This test which is used to detect prefrontal cortex lesions classically consists of discovering the principle according to which a deck of cards must be sorted (Grant and Berg 1948; Milner 1963). The cards bear geometric figures of different shapes (triangle, star, cross or circle), color (green, red, blue or yellow) and number (1, 2, 3 or 4 figures). Four reference cards are permanently placed in front of the subject. The subject has another deck of cards called the response cards. He is asked to match each response card successively with one of the four reference cards. After each response, he is told whether this is correct or not. The subject tries to achieve the maximum of correct responses. The rule will, for example, be sorting according to color. Once the subject is systematically successful in this, the rule is changed, for example from color to shape. The subject must understand that the rule has changed and discover the new rule (Fig. 5).

model includes four clusters of intention neurons. Each code for the choice of a particular reference card, and activation of one of them excludes activation of the others. The intention is converted into an output command when an external "go" signal is received. Finally, like the previous model, this model includes clusters of rule-coding neurons which play a critical role in the performance of the test. Indeed, they modulate the connections between memory clusters and intention clusters according to a defined category (color, shape, number, etc.) and their activity varies with time during learning since each cluster which is active at a given moment inhibits the others. The organism uses them to test "hypotheses" of rules of behavior and selects a particular rule by interpreting a reinforcement signal. In fact, the network has been modelled in such a way that each incorrect rule leads to punishment which, as in the previous model, destabilizes all the rule-coding neuron clusters so that they fluctuate in time and serve as the "generator of diversity."

Another novelty of the model is the differentiation of a "cluster of error neurons" which project and modulate the connections with rule-coding neuron clusters. The activity of error neurons is itself governed by reward signals so that a negative reward leads to short-term depression of excitatory connections in clusters of active rule-coding neurons. A molecular embodiment of this effect is the allosteric regulation of postsynaptic receptor desensitization of the type described previously. This depression is spontaneously reversible and the speed of recovery is a crucial parameter which determines the memory range of the generator of diversity. If this speed is fast, the cluster of rule-coding neurons which has just been eliminated immediately enters again into the generator of diversity; it is a [random] machine. If the recovery speed is slow, a [random + context] machine is obtained which retains only the rule that has just been eliminated. Finally, when this speed is very slow, recovery extends over several consecutive tests and the network memorizes all the rules which have failed. It then behaves like a [random + memory] machine. The most original feature of the new model is the "auto-evaluation loop" which short-circuits the reward input from the exterior. This allows endogenous activation by intention clusters of error clusters, the efficacy of which is changed according to a classical Hebb's scheme. When a negative reward is received, the error neurons are activated and the connection linking intention clusters which are active at that moment with error clusters is reinforced. This intention is labelled as incorrect. Due to the persistence of activity in the error neurons, a new rule is tested within the rule-coding layer. This new rule is applied to the memorized features of the preceding cue, which produces a new distribution of intention cluster activity. If this distribution is identical to the previous one, the rule is rejected because the activity of the error cluster is maintained by potentiation of the intention/error connection, which prevents stabilization of the new rule. The "internal evaluation" of rules sequence is pursued until a correct rule is found.

Simulation of networks possessing auto-evaluation and memory shows a single trial percentage success rate much higher than that of the [random + memory] machine (98.4% versus 39.8%). Similarly, a network with an auto-evaluation loop but no memory is more successful than the [random + context] machine (Fig. 6).

Lesioning of the error cluster leads to slowing of learning and an increase in perseverations similar to those observed in frontal patients (see above). The inertia of the generator of diversity becomes very large. As in the case of the simple network, lesioning of rule-coding clusters interferes with the acquisition of a "systematic" rule of behavior. Lesioning of the auto-evaluation loop has no major qualitative effect on the behavior of the organism except for a loss of ability to reason, which significantly slows the learning process. However, it might offer a formal explanation of the "sociopathic" behavior resulting from ventromedian lesions of the frontal cortex (Damasio et al. 1991). Damasio et al. (1990, see this volume) consider that this deficit is due to the inability to activate somatic states linked to the punishment or reward which the subject has experienced in association with specific social situations and which must be reactivated in connection with the anticipated result of a possible response. Injury to the intention/error connection might, according to our scheme, be the origin of this type of syndrome, evidently within a context both verbally and socially richer than that which served for modelling.

Conclusion

The two proposed formal models of the neuron network take into account the characteristic functional abilities of the prefrontal cortex: success in various delayed response tasks and in the Wisconsin card sorting test. They are based on principles of molecular, cellular and histological architecture that are plausible at the neurobiological level. These models are extremely simple and might even appear simplistic to cerebral cortex specialists. Nevertheless, they provide several original and specific predictions able to delineate novel experimental tests. One bears on the existence of "rule-coding neurons," the activity state of which varies randomly during the learning period until a rule of behavior is selected. Another concerns the mechanism, or mechanisms, of reinforcement by "error neurons." On the one hand their activity is regulated by that of neurons coding for motor intentions, and on the other hand they exert a regulatory action on rule-coding neuron clusters.

At a more general level, the induction of rule by trial and error followed by selection integrates perfectly with evolutionary epistemology (Darwin 1859; Poincare 1913; Popper 1966; Changeux et al. 1973; Campbell 1974; Edelman 1978; Changeux 1983; Changeux and Dehaene 1989; Dehaene and Changeux 1991) and illustrates the concept of "mental Darwinism" (Changeux and Dehaene 1989; see also Campbell 1974). In this context, clusters of rule-coding neurons would constitute the "generator of diversity." Memorization by selection may be considered as a homologue of "amplification" since the organism will re-use the memorized trace repeatedly in its subsequent behaviors.

The models also illustrate the precise contribution of hierarchical levels of network architecture to defined behaviors and particularly:

1. the ability to generalize a rule acquired for a particular cue to an entire class of cues, or systematicity (Dehaene and Changeux 1989; Fodor and Pylyshyn 1988);

2. the ability to "memorize" rules which have already been tested on the outside world; and
3. the ability to evaluate new rules in a tacit manner by internal auto-evaluation which may be taken as a very simple form of "reasoning" (Dehaene and Changeux 1991).

Finally, these models and their simulation show how some elementary components of the network (e.g., allosteric receptors, synaptic triads) can introduce constraints into higher cognitive functions ("bottom-up" regulation) (see Goldman-Rakic (1990) for the demonstration of synaptic triads with dopaminergic terminals in the prefrontal cortex). They also illustrate how a global process of interaction with the outside world, such as reward or reinforcement, can govern regulation at a more elementary level, such as the regulation of conformational transitions of allosteric receptors ("top-down" regulation). Last of all, they offer a specific illustration of the interdependence between levels of organization which confer structural coherence and functional integration on the system.

References

Amit DJ (1989) Modeling brain functions. Cambridge University Press, Cambridge

Batuev AS, Orlov AA, Pirogov AA (1981) Short-term spatio-temporal memory and cortical unit reactions in the monkey. Acta Physiol Hung. 58:207–216

Campbell DT (1974) Evolutionary epistomology. In: Schilpp PA (ed) The philosophy of Karl Popper. La Salle, Open Court

Changeux JP (1983) L'Homme neuronal. Fayard, Paris; English edition: Neuronal man, Pantheon New York

Changeux JP (1988) Molécule et mémoire. Bedou, Gordes

Changeux JP, Courrege P, Danchin A (1973) A theory of the epigenesis of neural networks by selective stabilization of synapses. Proc Natl Acad Sci USA 70:2974–2978

Changeux JP, Dehaene S (1989) Neuronal models of cognitive functions. Cognition 33:63–109

Changeux JP, Heidmann T (1987) Allosteric receptors and molecular models of learning. In: Edelman G, Gall WE, Cowan WM (eds) Synaptic Function. John Wiley, New York, pp 549–601

Damasio AR, Tranel D, Damasio H (1991) Somatic markers and the guidance of behavior: Theory and preliminary testing. In: Levin HS, Eisenberg HM, Benton AL (eds) Frontal Lobe Function and Dysfunction. Oxford University Press, New York, pp 217–229

Darwin C (1859) On the origin of species. London: Murray

Dehaene S, Changeux JP (1989) A simple model of prefrontal cortex function in delayed-response tasks, J Cognitive Neurosci 1:244–261

Dehaene S, Changeux JP (1991) The Wisconsin card sorting test: theoretical analysis and simulation of a reasoning task in a model neuronal network. Cerebral Cortex 1:62–79

Dehaene S, Changeux JP, Nadal JP (1987) Neural networks that learn temporal sequences by selection. Proc Natl Acad Sci USA 84:2727–2731

Diamond A (1985) The development of the ability to use recall to guide action, as indicated by infant's performance on AB. Child Develop 56:868–883

Diamond A (1988) Differences between adult and infant cognition: is the crucial variable presence or absence of language? In: Weiskrantz L (ed) Thought without language. Clarendon Press, Oxford

Edelman GM (1978) Group selection and phasic reentrant signaling: a theory of higher brain function. In: Edelman GM, Mountcastle VB (eds) The mindful brain: cortical organization and the group-selective theory of high brain function. MIT Press, Cambridge, pp 51–100

Fodor JA, Pylyshyn ZW (1988) Connectionism an cognitive architecture: A critical analysis.

Cognition 28:3–71

Fuster JM (1973) Unit activity in prefrontal cortex during delayed-response performance: Neuronal correlates of transient memory. J Neurophysiol 36:61–78

Fuster JM (1984) Electrophysiology of the prefrontal cortex. Trends Neurosci 1:408–414

Fuster JM (1989) The prefrontal cortex (2nd edition). Raven Press, New York

Funahashi S, Chafee MV, Goldman-Rakic P (1993) Prefrontal neuronal activity in rhesus monkeys performing a delayed anti-saccade task. Nature 365:753–756

Fuxe K, Agnati L (1991) Volume transmission in the brain: new aspects for electrical and chemical communication. Raven, New York

Goldman-Rakic P (1987) Circuitry of the primate prefrontal cortex and the regulation of behavior by representational knowledge. In: Mountcastle V, Plum KF (eds) The nervous system: Higher functions of the brain, Vol 5, Handbook of Physiology. American Physiological Society, Washington, DC

Goldman-Rakic PS (1990) Prog. Brain Res 85:325–335

Grant DA, Berg EA (1948) A behavioral analysis of degree of reinforcement and ease of shifting to new responses in a Weigl-type card-sorting problem. J Exp Psych 38:404–411

Heidmann T, Changeux JP (1982) Un modèle moléculaire de régulation d'efficacité d'une, synapse chimique au niveau postsynaptique. CR Acad Sci Paris, série 3, 295:665–670

Jacob F (1970) La logique du vivant. Gallimard, Paris

Kubota K, Niki H (1971) Prefrontal cortical unit activity and delayed alternation performance in monkeys. J Neurophysiol 34:337–347

Kubota K, Komatsu H (1985) Neuron activities of monkey prefrontal cortex during the learning of visual discrimination tasks with go-no go performances. Neurosci Res 3:106–129

Marr D (1982) Vision. Freeman, San Francisco

McCulloch WS, Pitts W (1943) A logical calculus of the ideas imminent in nervous activity. Bull Math Biophys 5:115–137

Milner B (1963) Effects of brain lesions on card sorting. Arch Neurol 9:90–100

Mountcastle VB (1978) An organizing principle for cerebral function: the unit module and the distributed system. In: Edelman GM, Mountcastle VB (eds) The mindful brain. The MIT Press, Cambridge

Nauta WJH (1971) The problem of the frontal lobe: a reinterpretation. J Psych Res 8:167–187

Newell A (1982) The knowledge level. Artificial Intelligence 18:87–127

Niki H (1974) Differential activity of prefrontal units during right and left delayed response trials. Brain Res 70:346–349

Niki H (1975) Differential activity of prefrontal units during right and left delayed response trials. In: Kawai M, Ehara A, Kawamura S (eds) Symposia of the Fifth Congress of International Primatological Society, Kondos, Japan Science Press, Tokyo, pp 475–486

Piaget J (1954) The construction of reality in the child. Basic Books, New York

Poincare H (1913) Science et Méthode. Flammarion, Paris

Popper KR (1963) Conjectures and refutations. Basic Books, New York

Popper KR (1966) Of clouds and clocks: an approach to the problem of rationality and the freedom of man. Washington University Press, St. Louis, Missouri

Rosenkilde E, Bauer CE, Fuster JM (1981) Single cell activity in ventral prefrontal cortex of behaving monkeys. Brain Res 209:375–394

Shallice T (1982) Specific impairments of planning. Phil Trans Royal Soc London B 298:199–209

Teuber HL (1964) The riddle of frontal lobe function in man. In: Warren JM, Akert K (eds) The frontal granular cortex and behavior. McGraw-Hill, New York, pp 410–477

Teuber HL (1972) Unity and diversity of frontal lobe functions. Acta Neurobiol Exp (Warsz.) 32:615–656

Watanabe M (1986a) Prefrontal unit activity during delayed conditional Go/No-Go discrimination in the monkey. II. Relation to Go and No-Go responses. Brain Res 382:15–27

Watanabe M (1986b) Prefrontal unit activity during delayed conditional discriminations in the monkey. Brain Res 225:51–65

Williams GV, Goldman-Rakic PS (1995) Modulations of memory fields by dopamine D, receptors in prefrontal cortex. Nature 376:572–575

Wilson FA, Scalaidhe SP, Goldman-Rakic P (1993) Disjociators of object and spatial processing domains in primate prefrontal cortex. Science 260:1955–1958

The Biological Causes of Irrationality

N.S. Sutherland

Introduction

1. Which is more dangerous, cycling or riding the Big Wheel?
2. Are there more words that begin with "k" than words that have "k" as the third letter?
3. If you are bored stiff by the first act of a play, should you see the second act in order "to get your money's worth"?
4. Are you a better than average driver?

The majority of people answer these questions incorrectly, except for the last one, which 40% of people must answer wrong since 90% of motorists think they are better than average drivers.

Everyone is irrational in one way or another, as I have tried to show in a recent book (Sutherland 1992), which lists about 100 different kinds of irrational behaviour. Only a few can be mentioned here. For full documentation of the phenomena described below, the reader should refer to my book, which cites the relevant experiments. I am indebted to others for the experimental findings, but the speculations on the biological origins of irrationality are my own.

It is important to be clear what constitutes irrationality; one must start by defining rationality. A rational decision is one that is most likely to lead to the end in view, given the knowledge that is available. An irrational decision is one that departs from this definition. Even rational decisions may not achieve their ends. If someone offers to bet you a pound to a penny that a toss of a coin will come down heads, it is rational to accept the bet, but you may lose money instead of gaining it. The uncertainty of human life means that almost all decisions are based on the balance of probabilities.

In classifying a decision as rational or irrational, some caution is needed. Several different ends may be relevant to a given decision and they may conflict. Unless a person has a clear hierarchy of the ends he wishes to pursue, it may be impossible to decide whether a given decision is rational. You may loathe taking exercise, but wish to feel fit. The question "To jog or not to jog?" can only be rationally answered if you can put a value on the two incompatible ends (as well as estimating how much fitter you will be if you jog). Moreover, as we will see, taking

Experimental Psychology, Biology Building, University of Sussex, Falmer, Brighton BN1 9QG, UK

A.R. Damasio et al. (Eds.)
Neurobiology of Decision-Making
© Springer-Verlag Berlin Heidelberg 1996

rational decisions is time-consuming and requires hard thought, which most people find unpleasant.

In most situations in everyday life, decisions are about matters that are so trivial that it is not worth devoting the time and thought needed to optimise them. But much hangs on certain personal decisions, such as buying a house, getting married or having children, and few people systematically think about the pros and cons. Darwin was an exception, for before marrying he carefully listed the points in favour and against. Moreover, the decisions taken by doctors, generals, engineers and other experts have important consequences. As has been repeatedly shown, experts are often highly irrational; they fall for the same fallacies as the man in the street. Finally, the exercise of rationality in everyday life does not affect my argument, for everyone would agree that the examples of bad decision-making that I give are irrational.

Since one can only justify an end in terms of a higher end, in the last analysis ends cannot be rational. It is generally assumed that all the ends we select are ultimately based on biological instincts, although the ways in which we follow those instincts are modifiable by experience. I will try to show that much if not all irrationality stems from the operation of primitive instincts and of features of the brain that are not adapted to present day conditions. Instincts often operate through mechanisms that no longer fulfill their original biological function. Sexual desire is a case in point. It is presumably based on the intense pleasure of copulation, but nowadays we can have that pleasure without the, for many, tedious necessity of having children. Similarly, breathing is regulated by the level of carbon dioxide in the blood. Normally this results in sufficient oxygen being inhaled, but the mechanism fails at great height. Pilots in open cockpits and without oxygen masks used to faint before they realised that anything was wrong.

Although sociobiologists have tried to account for human behaviour in terms of innate drives, there is a particularly powerful drive that is rarely mentioned and whose neurophysiological underpinnings are completely unknown. That drive is curiosity and the wish to master and understand the environment. Curiosity is present in every species of mammal in which it has been investigated, and it is almost entirely responsible for the whole of human culture as we know it. It can be used to explain the addiction of some people to crossword puzzles, the businessman's drive to accumulate more money, even though he has more than sufficient to meet all his other needs, and the activities of pure scientists. The survival value of exploring and mastering one's environment is obvious.

As a note of caution, it is difficult to explain all human activity in terms of drives that evolved in prehistoric times. What are we to make of a man who devotes himself to the welfare of people far removed from him, for example, by trying to alleviate famine in Ethiopia, while behaving abominably to his kith and kin, as so many do-gooders appear to do? The standard sociobiological explanation of altruism does not apply. He is not promoting his own genes by helping close kin and he is not looking for reciprocal benefits.

Social Pressures

People are highly social animals. If we did not have a drive to co-operate with and to be liked by our fellows, society would fall apart. Few people are capable of surviving on their own, and the more civilization advances, the more dependent each of us becomes on the skills of others. The social drive can, however, result in alarming mistakes. If a group of stooges – that is people in league with the experimenter – deliberately misjudge the lengths of lines in the presence of a subject who believes the stooges are also genuine subjects, most real subjects also misjudge the lines' lengths (Asch 1946).

The tendency to agree with others in order to please them can lead to irrational beliefs and decisions. If a group holds a common view, its members try to gain prestige by producing arguments in favour of that view and by outdoing one another in the strength with which they assert their belief in it. The result is a runaway process, not unlike the evolution of the peacock's tail, in which the group as a whole comes to have stronger views than any held by its individual members before they joined the group. For example, French schoolboys interviewed individually had a favourable view of de Gaulle, but after discussing him in a group, they formed even more favourable views (Moscovici and Personnaz 1969). In general, groups have more extreme views than individuals and they take riskier decisions; this cannot be rational (Kogan and Wallach 1964).

Unfortunately, it is impossible to feel proud of belonging to an in-group without despising out-groups. In order to boost the value of their own group, people denigrate and often come to hate out-groups. In a famous experiment, Sherif (1966) showed this tendency at work among boys at a holiday camp. They were divided into two groups with former friends assigned as far as possible to separate groups. Nevertheless, the rivalry between the groups became intense, leading to bullying and hatred. In addition, the in-group phenomenon has led to much prejudiced and irrational stereotyping and has been responsible for cruelty on a massive scale. It cannot be rational to persecute people merely because their religious beliefs are different from one's own.

Dominance Hierarchies

The irrationality produced by the wish to belong to a group is exacerbated by the tendency to form dominance hierarchies. It is likely that we have inherited a drive to become leaders, and if we fail, to be subservient to those who are. This can have disastrous effects in small groups such as committees, in which the other members of the group are driven to support the leader's opinions. By producing new arguments in favour of his views and suppressing counter-arguments, the group members increase the strength with which the leader holds his opinions. The result is extreme and irrational decision making. It was the respect for authority that led 75% of randomly picked American citizens to give what they thought were possibly lethal shocks to a stooge who was prancing around in simulated agony. In this famous experiment, conducted by Stanley Milgram (1974), the subjects presumably regarded him as an authority to whom obedience was due, for the Americans, unlike the English, hold professors in high esteem. This motive operates with adverse effects in many other situations. Junior doctors are afraid to tell a consultant that he is making a mistake; other aircrew are afraid to intervene when a senior pilot is clearly making an error. The stewardesses on the flight that crashed recently on a motorway in Britain because the pilot had shut down the wrong engine were well aware that it was the other engine that was on fire, but did not dare tell him of his error. In these situations, as in many others, more than one motive is sometimes at work, and the junior doctor may fail to contradict his consultant because the consultant has considerable power over his career. Nevertheless, from the point of view of society as a whole, the organisation of most institutions is irrational, for it promotes self-seeking behaviour in the members rather than behaviour that will secure the ends of the particular institution.

Emotional Effects

A further evolutionary reason for irrational behaviour may be that our ancestors often had to take immediate decisions without time for thought. When confronted by a predator, it is surely better to climb a non-optimal tree than to be eaten while weighing the respective merits of different trees. Strong emotion leads to the perseverance of whatever is the strongest habit and to a narrowing of attention that results in less obvious actions not being considered. Clarke Hull (1943), a much underestimated behaviourist, was the first to formulate this idea. He held that behaviour was governed by, among other things, the product of "drive strength" and "habit strength." If drive is high, the absolute difference between the tendency to perform the habit with highest strength and the tendency to perform weaker habits is increased. Behaviours that have low habit strength will therefore not have a chance to appear. To give an example from everyday life of the effects of strong emotion, upon losing their wallet most people will frantically search for it over and over again in the most obvious place in which they might have left it. They do not stop to consider when they last had it; neither do they carry out a systematic search in the places they have visited since.

Drives are governed not only by internal factors but by external ones; in particular, the prospect of a large reward heightens the drive to obtain it. Hence, behaviour becomes much less flexible when large rewards are offered. Although the pernicious influence of rewards on thinking has been demonstrated in dozens of experiments (e.g., Glucksberg 1962), society acts irrationally by offering prizes ranging from that for the schoolboy who is top of the class to the Nobel prize for eminent scientists.

It is well known that animals and people tend to make responses that lead to immediate reward rather than responses that lead to a delayed but larger reward. If young children are offered a choice between one chocolate now and several later on, they choose the immediate reward. In organisms that cannot systematically plan for the future, this makes good sense. But, although people can make such plans, they often continue to prefer a short-term gain to larger long-term gains. They overeat, they drink too much, and they smoke. Our reward system has not adapted to our capacity to think about the future.

The Maintenance of Beliefs

One of the commonest types of irrationality arises from the desire to be right. It leads people to maintain courses of action and opinions in the face of overwhelming evidence that they are wrong. Einstein spent many fruitless years trying to prove that the physical world was a deterministic system. In order to maintain their beliefs, people unconsciously use a variety of strategems. They refuse to look for contradictory evidence. If you have bought a new car, you read advertisements on that make rather than ones on other makes; you are seeking evidence that you have taken the right decision. Wason (1960) performed an ingenious experiment demonstrating this tendency. Subjects were given three numbers, were told that they obeyed a rule and were asked to formulate the rule governing the sequence. They were allowed to choose further sequences of three numbers and, for each sequence, were told whether it obeyed the rule. The subjects formed hypotheses, but to test them they tended to choose only further sets of numbers that would confirm them. For example, a subject shown "2, 4, 6" as the first sequence, might decide that the rule was "Even numbers ascending in twos" and would pick sets likely to confirm it such as "20, 22, 24", "8, 10, 12" rather than ones like "3, 7, 9" or "6, 4, 2" that could disconfirm the hypothesis. As a result the correct rule – "Any three numbers in ascending order" – was very hard to reach. Many if not most scientists make the same mistake. Having formulated a theory, they attempt to confirm it by performing experiments that are likely to do so. Few scientists carry out experiments that they feel are likely to disconfirm their own theories, though they are of course keen to obtain results that will disprove the theories of others.

The cause of this kind of error is not easy to establish. It may be linked to mental laziness, which the Gestalt psychologists, seeking to raise their status by borrowing from physics, called "the principle of least action." Just as we conserve physical energy, so presumably we conserve mental energy, that is, we do not spend more time thinking about something than is necessary. But to change one's opinions radically involves a great deal of mental effort. The evidence that led to the wrong view has to be resifted and explained away; it is easier simply to discard new evidence. It is something of a puzzle that people find it so difficult to think hard about a problem for any length of time. After all, the energy consumed by the brain in hard thought cannot be much more than the energy used when we are merely daydreaming. A problem that is difficult to solve cannot be solved quickly, and failure to solve it is likely to produce frustration, an emotion known to be aversive in all vertebrates. It may be that the inability to bear frustration is what makes prolonged thinking so difficult. Our ancestors presumably did not need much mental tenacity; if one flint could not be readily sharpened it was better to give up and try another.

A second possible biological cause for the difficulty in giving up beliefs lies in the organization of the brain, parts of which are probably connectionist networks. If an opinion is represented in such a network, any alteration of the opinion would involve a massive restructing of the network's connectivity. As far as I know, no one has proposed a mechanism that would account for a sudden and drastic change in output (representing a change of mind) in a connectionist system.

A further reason for the persistence of false beliefs may be the preservation of self-respect. In a social group it is obviously beneficial to be respected by others; at the extreme, this leads to being dominant in the dominance hierarchy. Because we are capable of self-reflection, we can respect ourselves just as others may respect us. Part of self-respect surely comes from being right; hence it is difficult to admit errors even to ourselves. Self-respect also leads to other errors, for example, the massive overconfidence that people have been shown to have about their own judgements (Lichenstein et al. 1977).

Availability and Connectionism

A further kind of irrationality, often demonstrated, may play a role in the maintenance of existing beliefs. It is the availability heuristic: people often base judgements on what is most available to their minds. Most people believe there are more words that begin with "k" than words that have "k" as a third letter. Because words are organised in memory by their initial letter (or phoneme), it is easier to retrieve words beginning with "k" than words with "k" in a later position. Emotional impact can also determine saliency. Most people believe it is less safe to ride the Big Dipper than to bicycle for the same length of time. In fact cycling in a town is 40 times as dangerous, but accidents in Big Dippers are more dramatic. The frequency with which an event has recently occurred also influences judgement. Doctors who have by chance encountered a particular non-infectious illness several times within a brief period are more likely to diagnose the same illness for some time thereafter.

The availability error is not caused by the effects of primitive drives, but it might be explained in terms of connectionist systems, which are likely to be heavily influenced by the most salient idea, whose representation will have the strongest connections in the network. Moreover, mental laziness may play a part. It is easier to use the first thing that comes to mind than to rack one's brain for less obvious but possibly more relevant ideas.

It is likely that availability is yet another reason for our reluctance to change our opinions. We will have rehearsed arguments for our own position and will have found counter-arguments for anything that goes against it. These arguments will be available and will make it difficult to abandon beliefs. This idea has been substantiated in an experiment in which subjects were told of two firemen, one of whom took risks while the other was very cautious. Half the subjects were told that the venturous fireman was a better fireman than the cautious one, the other half were told the opposite. Some of the subjects were asked to think up reasons why one fireman was good and the other bad. All of them were then told that the two firemen did not exist; they were pure inventions of the experimenter. The subjects who had been asked to think of reasons why one fireman was good and the other bad stuck much more firmly than the others to the belief originally implanted by the experimenter (Nisbett and Ross 1980).

Another error that may be due to availability is ignoring the base rate. This effect has been repeatedly demonstrated in experimental studies, of which the best known is described by Tversky and Kahneman (1978). Subjects were told that in a certain city there are two cab companies: the Blue Cabs, which own 85% of the cabs, and the Green Cabs, which own 15%. A cab is involved in a hit-and-run accident and a witness says she thought it was a green one. Tests were made and it was found she could correctly identify the colour of the cab 80% of the time in the lighting conditions under which the accident took place; 20% of the time she mistakenly thought a blue cab was green or a green cab blue. The question posed was whether the cab in the accident is more likely to have been blue or green. When tested, the majority of subjects reply "green," but they were wrong. Although the woman's judgement is usually accurate, there are far more blue cabs than green. The probability of her having seen a blue cab (0.85) and having thought it was green (0.2) is $0.85 \times 0.2 = 0.17$, whereas the chance of her having seen a green cab (0.15) and judging it green (0.8) is $0.15 \times 0.8 = 0.12$ (these figures do not add to 1.0 because all her other possible judgements would be "blue"). The conditional probability of the cab being green is the probability that it is green when the witness says green divided by the probability of her saying green, which is $0.15/(0.17 + 0.15) = 0.4$. The cab is therefore more likely to be blue than green. The subjects' error is to pay too much attention to new evidence about an event (the woman's judgement) at the expense of paying sufficient attention to the general frequency of that event (the frequency of green cabs). The conditional information is more available than the a priori information (the base rate), possibly because the latter is more abstract.

Apart from contributing to the availability error, connectionist systems may well produce many other sloppy errors in everyday thinking. In one experiment (Tversky and Kahneman 1983), a description of a woman, Linda, was given. She was said to be bright, to have a social conscience and so on. Subjects were then asked whether it was more likely that she was a feminist or a bank teller. The subjects all agreed that she was more likely to be a feminist, but they also thought she was more likely to be a feminist bank teller than merely a bank teller. Since the class of bank tellers is larger than the class of feminist bank tellers, this cannot possibly be true. But the inclusion of the word "feminist" in the description "feminist bank teller" might arouse more direct associations with Linda in a connectionist system than "bank teller" on its own; hence the error.

Mistaken Consistency

Allied to the perseverance of false beliefs is the inability to tolerate seeming inconsistencies. Here again connectionist networks and self-respect probably play a role. It has repeatedly been shown that, when subjects are forced to make a choice between two options, they increase the value placed on the option chosen. If you buy a house with a small dining room that was previously seen as poky, it is now seen as cosy. You are reassuring yourself that you have made the right decision.

The dislike of inconsistency also gives rise to the "halo effect." If someone has a highly salient good trait, such as being exceptionally handsome or pretty, his or her other traits are judged by others to be much better on average than they in fact are. Mental laziness may also play a part: it is simpler to regard someone as wholly good (or wholly bad) than to evaluate all his different characteristics one by one. This mechanism also plays a role in stereotyping. Stereotypes may contain elements of truth, but when we meet a member of the stereotyped class it is easier to assume that he or she has all the stereotypical characteristics than to look for exceptions.

Bias caused by preconceptions, itself tied to the attempt at consistency, plays a large role in thought. For example, in Britain Mrs. Thatcher's government wanted to reduce grants given to students. It was argued that, since university students earn more money in latter life than people who have not been to university, it was unfair to pay their grants out of taxes contributed by everyone. The flaw in the argument is obvious. University students are on average more intelligent and come from better homes than those who do not go to university; such privileged people might well earn more than others, regardless of whether or not they receive a university education.

There are two further errors with which everyone is familiar that are caused by misplaced consistency. The first is the sunk costs error. You go to a play, are bored stiff, but do not leave after the interval because you want to get your "money's worth." So as well as losing the price of a ticket you have to suffer an extra hour of boredom. People cannot admit that they have made a mistake by abandoning a project in which they have invested, even when it is clearly in their best interest to do so. A related error can be illustrated by the case of someone who buys a ticket for a play that he very much wants to see, but loses the ticket. He refuses to buy another one, even if he can afford it, on the principle that he does not want to pay for the same play twice. He has failed to realise that nothing he can do will recover the cost of the first ticket. The past is the past. Assuming he still wants to see the play, it will cost him exactly what he was originally prepared to spend. Connectionist systems have exhibited some interesting and surprising forms of learning, but the very fact that such systems tend to settle into a state of maximum consistency may make them inefficient at reasoning.

Curiosity and Mastery

The innate drive of seeking to master the environment may be responsible for some irrational judgements. We often find connections between events where

	DISEASE	NO DISEASE
SYMPTOM	37	33
NO SYMPTOM	17	13

Fig. 1. The distribution of types of case history presented on cards to nurses (after Smedslund 1963)

none exists. In one experiment (Smedslund 1963), nurses were shown cards recording case histories. There were four kinds of cases: cases where a given disease was present with a given symptom, cases where the disease was present but not the symptom, cases where the disease was absent and the symptom present and cases where neither disease nor symptom was present. The distribution of the four types of case over a hundred cards in shown in Figure 1. Although there is clearly no association between the disease and the symptom, 85% of the nurses believed that the symptom was associated with the disease. Similar errors have been found in many other experiments. It may be said that the subjects were looking at the cards one by one and thus could not draw up a two-by-two table, inspection of which would have shown that there was no correlation between the symptom and the disease. But this does not explain why the mistake made is always that of associating the two positive events (disease present and symptom present). Our curiosity and desire for mastery may make us look too hard for associations between events. In addition it is likely that people pay too little attention to the absence of an event because it is not so available: this would cause people not to take into account the bottom right hand cell of the figure, where neither event is present.

Statistical Reasoning

There are of course many errors of thinking and decision-making that cannot be explained in biological or evolutionary terms. In particular there is a vast class of mistakes that arises either from people's ignorance of probability theory and statistics or from their failure to use their knowledge of these subjects in everyday reasoning. Two examples must suffice. Kahneman and Tversky (1973) found that, in the Israeli air force, pilot trainers complained to their superior officer that if a trainee pilot flew particularly well one day, they would praise him and he almost always flew less well the next day. On the other hand, when they blamed a trainee for flying badly, he would usually fly better the following day. The trainers suggested they should abandon the use of praise. They had failed to see that the phenomenon they were describing was simply an example of regression to the mean. Pilot performance is determined by many chance factors. On most days, therefore, pilots will fly at about their average level of proficiency, so that a very good or very bad day is likely to be followed by a more or less average day.

In a second example, many people think that if you toss a coin six times you are more likely to get the sequence THHTHT than the sequence TTTTTT (where 'H' stands for heads and "T" for tails). The first sequence is hard to distinguish from most other random sequences and therefore seems to people more likely, but of course both sequences occur with the same probability, $(1/2)^6$ or 1/64.

Unless people are prepared to undergo the rigors of doing some arithmetic, they are likely to be wildly wrong. For example, it has been shown that in estimating a probability that is based on the probability of occurrence of a series of independent events, people's estimates are far too low. Few people realise that in an accumulator bet, where each horse has a one in ten chance of being first at the post in each race, the chance of winning the bet is one in a thousand. Unless they do the formal multiplication their estimates of the probability are far too high. Correspondingly, if there are a large number of factors, each with a low probability and each of which, if it occurred, could cause an event (such as a plane crash), people's estimates are much too low. In both cases the estimates stick too closely to the individual values of the probabilities.

A knowledge of probability theory and statistics reduces some of the errors described here, including ones that are common in everyday life, for example, the sunk costs error. But few people take the trouble to learn these subjects even at an elementary level. For whatever reason the human brain is sloppy. Its sloppiness may sometimes lead to remarkable insights at the cost of many false starts, but rigorous thinking depends largely on the use of symbols and on our ability to externalise those symbols on paper. The small size of working memory prevents us from doing complicated symbol manipulation in our heads. Compare the difficulty we have in manipulating formal symbols with the ease with which in vision we process a scene, recognising the objects within it. The computations undertaken by the visual system involve symbols (for example, the firing of a motion detecting cell or a "line detector"), but the mechanism for handling symbols in the visual system has evolved over millions of years and is completely hidden from consciousness. Accurate visual perception occurs with remarkable ease, yet the workings of the visual system are more complex than the thinking of an Einstein. In terms of evolution, there has been little time (perhaps 10,000 years) to develop the apparatus for conscious symbol manipulation (except for the symbols of a natural language), and even then there has probably been little or no evolutionary pressure. In fact, what requires explanation is not why most people are poor mathematicians, but why some are such good ones. Despite the many extraordinary intuitions of scientists, it is almost certainly true that most intuitive judgements are wrong, though this can only be proven when one can substitute a formal system for them. It has been remarked that intuition is the faculty that tells you you are right when you are wrong.

Indeed it has been shown (for a review, see Dawes 1988) that by correlating the past values of each of a set of predictors with the occurrence of a predicted type of event, it is possible to achieve predictions of the future occurrence of that type of event that are more accurate than those made by human experts in the domain. Here are some examples in which this has been found to be true (the type of expert with whom the statistical prediction is compared is shown in brackets): the extent to which people on parole will show good conduct or will violate their parole – three separate studies on over 3,000 parolees (psychologists and psychiatrists); pilot performance after training predicted before training (US Air Force personnel officers); adjustment to a reformatory (psychiatrists); job satisfaction in engineers predicted before they left college (counsellors); recidivism in criminals (physicians); suicide attempts in psychiatric patients (psychiatrists); amelioration of mental illness in schizophrenics (physicians); whether to classify a mental patient as psychotic or neurotic (psychiatrists and psychologists); the growth of corporations (securities analysts); and horses' performance at the races (tipsters).

Human experts cannot reach the best decisions by insight. The accuracy of their judgement is restricted by the small size of working memory, the inability to work with arithmetic symbols and even by variations in judgement caused by swings of mood. But there is a further act of irrationality; at least in medicine, even where there are statistical methods that are known to be more accurate than the experts, doctors usually refuse to use them. The drive for self-respect leads to an unwarranted confidence in their own judgements in the face of all the evidence.

Conclusion

I have tried to show that many errors of thought are caused by drives or emotions that are not adapted to manipulating the knowledge gained in a few thousand years of civilization. The relevant factors include: group pressures; dominance hierarchies; the narrowing of attention under emotion or stress; the mechanism governing the effects of reward, curiosity and the desire to master the environment; self-regard – itself a spinoff from the need to belong to a group; mental laziness – possibly produced by frustration; the small size of working memory; and the operation of connectionist systems in the brain. I have also called attention to two outstanding problems: why are people so mentally lazy and how are sudden changes of mind possible given the substrate of the nervous system as we know it?

I should end with two cautioning notes. First, none of what I have written conflicts with Damasio's theory of emotion (Damasio 1994). He has discovered some of its beneficial effects on cognition, whereas I have tried to show that it can also have detrimental effects, which are mainly caused by the mechanisms of the drive or emotion in question having failed to adapt to the culture in which we now live and, in particular, to the emergence of elaborate thought processes that can help us to determine the likely consequences of our actions even in the distant future. Second, my own explanations of irrational decisions do not conflict with the explanations in terms of cognition that are commonly given (see, for example, Dawes 1984; Kahneman et al. 1982; Nisbett and Ross 1980). The cognitive factors usually cited undoubtedly exist. I am merely arguing that many of them are determined by more fundamental biological factors, whether at a higher level (instincts) or at a lower level (connectionist systems). *Pax vobiscum.*

References

Asch S (1946) Forming impressions of personality. J Abnormal Social Psychol 41:258–290

Damasio AR (1994) Descartes' error. Emotion reasons and the human brain. Grosset/Putnam, New York

Dawes, RM (1988) Rational choice in an uncertain world. Orlando, Harcourt, Brace Jovanovich

Glucksberg S (1962) The influence of strength of drive on functional fixedness and perceptual recognition. J Exper Psychol 63:36–41

Hull CL (1943) Principles of behaviour. New York, Appleton-Century-Crofts

Kahneman D, Tversky A (1973) On the psychology of prediction. Psychol Rev 80:237–251

Kahneman D, Slovic P, Tversky A (1982) Judgment under uncertainty: heuristics and biases. Cambridge, Cambridge University Press

Kogan N, Wallach MA (1964) Risk taking: A study in cognition and personality. New York, Holt, Rinehart & Winston

Lichenstein S, Fischhoff B, Phillips LD (1977) Calibration of probabilities: The state of the art. In: Jungermann, H, de Zeeuw G (eds) Decision making and change in human affairs. Amsterdam, D. Reidel

Milgram S (1974) Obedience to authority: an experimental view. New York, Harper and Row

Moscovici S, Personnaz B (1969) Studies in social influence. V. Minority influence and conversion behaviour in a perceptual task. J Personality Social Psychol 12:125–135

Nisbett R, Ross L (1980) Human inference: strategies and shortcomings of social judgement. Englewood Cliffs, Prentice-Hall

Sherif M (1966) Group conflict and co-operation: their social psychology. London, Routledge and Kegan Paul

Smedslund J (1963) The concept of correlation in adults. Scand J Psychol 4:165–173

Sutherland S (1992) Irrationality: the enemy within. London, Constable

Tversky A, Kahneman D (1978) Causal schemata in judgements under uncertainty. In: Fishbein M (ed) Progress in social psychology. Hillsdale, NJ, Erlbaum

Tversky A, Kahneman D (1983) Extensional versus intuitive reasoning: The conjunction fallacy in probability judgement. Psychol Rev 90:293–315

Wason PC (1960) On the failure to eliminate hypotheses in a conceptual task. Quart J Exper Psychol 12:129–140

Neuropsychological Approaches to Reasoning and Decision-Making

R. Adolphs, D. Tranel, A. Bechara, H. Damasio, and A.R. Damasio

Abstract

How do people reason and decide? Patients with damage to the ventromedial frontal cortex help answer this question, since their lesion renders their choices in the real world irrational, i.e., not in their best interest. Our approach was to describe dysfunction in real life circumstances and then to attempt to analyze the components of this dysfunction with controlled laboratory manipulations, employing psychophysiological and neuropsychological methods. The results we report in this paper suggest that this group of patients is defective in an essential and specific component of reasoning, the ability to guide choice by feeling.

Introduction

Human Reasoning Theories

Human reasoning has traditionally been situated between two extremes. Some have claimed that the way we reason is similar to the way problems are solved in formal logic: reasoning is rule-based and content-insensitive (Rips 1983). Others have considered reasoning to be "associative": problems are compared to similar situations that have been encountered in the past, and reasoning is idiosyncratic with respect to content and context.

Most theories of human reasoning fall somewhere between these two positions (Cheng and Holyoak 1985; Cosmides and Tooby 1992; Gigerenzer and Hug 1992; Johnson-Laird and Byrne 1991; for review see Evans et al. 1993). Typically, reasoning is thought to make use of some rules, which may all be implicit. But reasoning is also thought to be sensitive to features other than the mere syntactic structure of the problem. Background knowledge, context, and problem content all appear to play a role in the strategies we deploy for reasoning. In particular, different strategies may be applied depending on the relevance of the problem and the goal of the person faced with it.

Department of Neurology, Division of Cognitive Neuroscience, The University of Iowa College of Medicine, Iowa City, IA 52242, USA

A.R. Damasio et al. (Eds.)
Neurobiology of Decision-Making
© Springer-Verlag Berlin Heidelberg 1996

We have recently proposed a framework for understanding human reasoning and decision-making that is informed by data from neuropsychology (Damasio et al. 1991; Damasio 1994). In our view, human reasoning incorporates mechanisms at many levels, ranging from those that perform basic body regulation to those that control complex strategies based on language. A novel component of this picture is that reason depends on the process of feeling and its underpinnings, and that feeling involves images that pertain to the state of the body. Our proposal stresses that reasoning is not disembodied, but instead uses biological information in order to guide decision-making through a complex space of possible options and outcomes.

The specific hypothesis we have put forth is known as the somatic marker hypothesis. This hypothesis proposes that decisions whose outcome could be potentially harmful, or potentially advantageous, and that are made in circumstances similar to previous experience, prompt a somatic response. This response involves autonomic, endocrine, visceral and musculoskeletal routes of expression, and is used to mark future outcomes that are important to the organism, and to signal their danger or advantage. Signalling proceeds in several ways: the somatic marker focuses attention on the situation and probably promotes working memory; and the valence of the feeling signified by the somatic marker signals the merit of the option-outcome ensemble. We may have a good or a bad feeling about something, but in either case the feeling alerts us as to the nature of the future facing us, and serves to guide our subsequent behavior.

It is also part of the hypothesis that the "somatic marker" does not need to be implemented in the body proper (via the "body loop") but can instead be directly engendered in somatosensory cortices (via the "as-if loop"). Either mode of "somatic" marking may be overt (we may be aware of it), or covert (processed below the level of conscious awareness). The reader is referred to A. Damasio (1994) for details on somatic markers, and to A. Damasio (1995) for details on mechanisms of emotion and feeling.

In our view, reasoning delineates a domain of cognition in which an organism must choose how to respond to a situation. Concepts such as "decision," "choice," "reason," and "rationality" are essentially linked to behavior. When an agent faces a situation, she must decide what to do next. Her decision/choice is mediated by the reasoning engaged. If the outcome of the reasoning, and the subsequent decision as evidenced in behavior, are adaptive (to the agent's advantage in the long run), the choice is rational (see Note 1). This view is different from the traditional account, in which human reasoning and choice are fraught with biases and errors, and hence are often irrational (Stich 1985; see also Manktelow and Over 1987). Some of the difference comes about for at least two reasons. First, most studies of human reasoning have measured performance on formal and artificial tasks, which do not necessarily correspond to how we make decisions in the real world. In fact, studies have found people's reasoning in the laboratory to differ substantially from their behavior in the real world (Ebbeson and Konecni 1980). Secondly, the motivation for our research is to discover what subjects are actually doing when they try to reason, rather than how their behavior differs from the predictions of a normative theory. When reasoning and decision-making are examined in an ethological context, much of human competence can be described as rational, in the sense that it is adaptive under the circumstances and under the constraints of human cognitive capacities (Evans 1993). Nonetheless, there is no question that some human reasoning, even in light of ethological descriptions, is irrational (Sutherland 1992). We also agree that examinations of the logical errors that subjects make can shed light on how they reason; but that is not our purpose in the experiments we report here. We compare performances among different groups of subjects, rather than compare a performance to what might be considered "correct" vis-a-vis some theory. In this framework, then, the choices that control subjects make are "normal", and the choices made by subjects with lesions of the ventromedial frontal cortex are defective compared to normal choices, even though normal choices themselves may be logically incorrect.

Studies using factor analysis strongly suggest that reasoning is a complex capacity that cannot be easily decomposed into a small number of simple factors (Carroll 1993, especially Chapter 6). Some theoretical treatments have gone so far as to suggest that reasoning, insofar as it draws on nearly all other psychological abilities, cannot even be studied (Fodor 1983). However, we take the view that reasoning is in fact methodologically modular, and that lesion studies in humans (Damasio and Damasio 1989) can shed some light on how human reasoning abilities are generated by large-scale neural systems.

Rationale of Experiments

Our neuropsychological studies focus on the contributions made to reasoning by sectors of the prefrontal cortex. A long history of studies suggests that this brain region is important in reasoning (Levin et al. 1991). Lesions of the prefrontal cortex in animals impair performance on many cognitive factors that are essential to successful reasoning (Fuster 1989; Passingham 1972; Kowalska et al. 1991; Voytko 1985; Wilson et al. 1993). The responses of neurons within this region also correlate with cognitive operations that are presumably required during reasoning (Fuster 1989; Goldman-Rakic 1990; Funahashi et al. 1993). The large increase in the size of the prefrontal cortex in the evolution of primates, and during their development, lend further support to the idea that the advanced reasoning capacities of higher primates and of humans are tied to the frontal lobes (e.g., Diamond and Goldman-Rakic 1989).

The prefrontal cortex consists of many different sectors (Fuster 1989; Pandya and Barnes 1987; H. Damasio, this volume). Although it is often difficult to distinguish their boundaries, a rough but robust division can be made between ventromedial sectors ("VM frontal cortex"), which include more poorly laminated paralimbic mesocortex (Morecraft et al. 1992), and dorsolateral sectors ("DL frontal cortex"), which show the well-developed lamination of isocortex, and whose connections more clearly situate them within sensori-motor neocortical networks (Goldman-Rakic 1988). While there are numerous further subdivisions within these sectors, and while ventromedial and dorsolateral cortices are heavily interconnected, the utility of this division is borne out both by connectivity (Barbas et al. 1991) and function (Rosenkilde 1979).

The somatic marker theory, discussed above, hypothesizes that somatic states are engaged in many instances of decision-making and reasoning. The function of these somatic states is to steer the decision-making process toward those outcomes that are advantageous for the subject, based on the subject's past experience with similar situations. This hypothesis was motivated by two findings: (1) lesions of the VM frontal cortex in man result in a profound inability to make successful decisions in real life, in the context of relatively spared memory, language and most other cognitive functions (Damasio et al. 1994; Eslinger and Damasio 1985); and (2) the VM frontal cortex is situated anatomically such that it can receive highly processed sensory information from all sensory modalities, and such that it can interact with neural systems that control skeletomotor, visceral and neuroendocrine effectors. To test the hypothesis, we have conducted a large number of studies with patients who have damage to the VM frontal cortex. In order to obtain clear evidence that could support or refute our somatic marker hypothesis, we chose subjects according to the following criteria: (1) they must have a lesion that includes sectors of the VM frontal cortex; (2) this lesion must be stable and contiguous; (3) the subjects must have been neurologically and psychiatrically normal prior to sustaining this lesion.

Psychophysiological Experiments

First we briefly summarize results of psychophysiological studies, which have been published in detail elsewhere (Damasio et al. 1990; Damasio et al. 1991; Tranel 1994; Tranel and Damasio 1994). We wanted to test the hypothesis that patients with bilateral damage to the VM frontal cortex will be defective in their ability to engage somatic states in response to stimuli with an emotionally complex meaning. Our reasoning was that the processing of stimuli with complex emotional significance would depend on the prior experiences subjects had with those stimuli, and that the VM frontal cortex would be an essential node in the reconstitution of somatic states that had been elicited by these stimuli on previous occasions.

The experiments measured a robust autonomic variable as one index of somatic state: the change in skin conductance (SCR) in response to a stimulus. Three groups of subjects were used: 1) neurologically and psychiatrically normal subjects; 2) subjects with lesions outside the frontal cortex; and 3) subjects with lesions of the VM frontal cortex. Subjects in group 3 all had bilateral lesions and all exhibited defects in decision-making in real life. Subjects were shown slides of two types: neutral slides (landscapes or abstract pictures) and emotionally significant target slides (scenes of nudity, social disaster, or mutilation). While all three groups of subjects showed robust SCRs to startling stimuli, such as a loud noise, or to behaviors that reliably elicit SCRs, such as a deep breath, the VM frontal group showed specific defects in response to emotionally significant stimuli (scenes of

Fig. 1. Skin conductance responses to visual stimuli. Subjects were shown slides (arrows) of either neutral stimuli or emotionally significant stimuli (nudes or social disasters, "T"). Skin conductance responses of a VM frontal subject are shown at the top; those of a brain-damaged control are shown at the bottom. The two traces are recordings from each hand

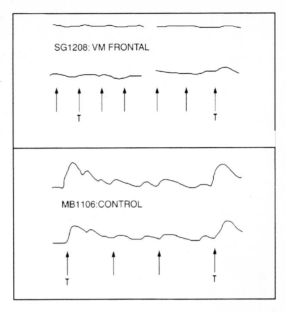

nudity, or of mutilation). Control groups showed larger SCRs to target stimuli than to neutral slides, whereas the VM frontal group failed to show significantly different SCR magnitudes between the two classes of stimuli (Fig. 1). These results suggest that VM frontal patients are defective in their ability to trigger somatic responses to stimuli with emotional meaning.

The Gambling Experiments

A second line of experiments investigated subjects' performance on a card-gambling task (Bechara et al. 1994). This task presents subjects with 4 decks of cards, and they are asked to pick a card from one deck at a time. Certain decks, unknown to the subject, are associated with a high probability of a large, immediate monetary reward and with a high probability of a large, delayed monetary loss. Other decks are associated with a low immediate monetary reward, and also a low risk of monetary loss. Subjects attempt to make as much money as possible by choosing sequentially from the decks; they are told how much money they have won or lost after each card that they have chosen. The probabilistic contingencies of the task have the consequence that correct responses cannot easily be computed overtly by the subjects, and subjects must rely instead on a "hunch" for the right response; this hunch is acquired as the subject gains experience and obtains feedback on the task. A normal subject's responses typically feature several choices from the high reward- high risk decks at the beginning of the experiment. Soon, the subject learns that these decks are not worth the risk, because sooner or later one loses more money than one has won. Later in the experiment, normal subjects invariably choose from the safer, low-income, low-risk decks. In the long run, this strategy allows the subject to win money overall.

Subjects with VM frontal lesions, however, do not show this switch in strategy. They invariably lose money on the task as a result of continuously choosing cards from the risky decks, even after they have had substantial experience with the decks, and have lost money on them. Interestingly, the VM frontal patients are quite aware that they are losing money, and some even figure out the fact that the decks from which they are choosing are likely to be more risky. None of this knowledge, however, appears to influence their abnormal behavior, and they continue to choose from risky decks despite continued losses.

To test the somatic marker theory explicitly, we measured an index of somatic state, skin conductance, while subjects were engaged in the task. We found that normal subjects show a SCR as they are deliberating a response in the task. This anticipatory SCR appears to be a component of a warning to subjects that they are about to make a risky choice. As a result, they tend not to choose cards on which they could potentially lose money in the long run. Whereas normal controls show large SCRs in anticipation of choosing a card from one of the risky decks, the patients with VM frontal lesions do not show these normal anticipatory SCRs (Bechara et al. in press). Despite their failure to trigger normal SCRs to the anticipation of a risky choice, ventromedial frontal subjects do show SCRs when they find out that they lost or won money (Fig. 2). Thus, the defect is not a general

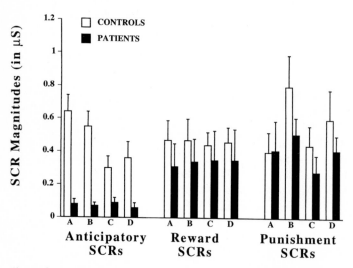

Fig. 2. Skin conductance responses while deliberating on a card-gambling task. Risky decks of cards, on which subjects can lose large sums of money, are decks A and B; safer decks, on which subjects win less money immediately, but make more in the long run, are decks C and D. Controls soon begin to show large skin conductance responses when about to choose from a risky deck, and avoid decks A and B on future occasions. However, VM frontal patients, despite normal skin conductance responses to actually winning or losing money on the cards ("punishment" and "reward"), do not show the anticipatory responses that the controls show. Consequently, they do not avoid the risky decks and end up losing money in the task

insensitivity to reward or punishment, but specifically a defect in using such reward or punishment in the future to guide decision-making. The VM frontal subjects are thus defective at using prior experience to trigger somatic states and to guide choices.

The Wason Selection Task

Another means to examine human reasoning strategies involves the Wason Selection Task (WST), the most popular experimental design for probing deductive reasoning (Wason 1966; Wason and Johnson-Laird 1972). The WST has been the subject of hundreds of studies, and has led to several current models of human reasoning. We briefly review the most robust findings from the WST that have been reported in the literature and discuss some current models. Then we present our own results with neurological populations, and argue that they support the somatic marker hypothesis.

The WST consists of a conditional statement, often presented in some context, and subjects must decide if the statement is really true. They do this by deciding which of four cards to turn over. All conditional statements are of the form "If P then Q", where P and Q stand for propositions. Each of the four cards denotes the four possible situations that could obtain with respect to the propositions P and Q. They are:

(1) P is true; Q is true (P&Q);
(2) P is true; Q is false (P&~Q);
(3) P is false, Q is true (~P&Q);
(4) P is false, Q is false (~P & ~Q).

One side of a card will say if P is true or false; the other side of that card will say if Q is true or false. Subjects see only one side of a card, and they must decide if turning the card over could tell them whether or not the conditional statement they are testing is true or false. Consider the following example (Wason and Shapiro 1971):

Conditional: "if you go to Chicago, then you take the car."

These four cards stand for the travels of four people. One side of a card gives the city they travelled to, the other side of a card tells how they got there.

Chicago	New York	Car	Plane

Which cards do you think are necessary to turn over in order to determine if the conditional statement is true or false? Surprisingly, it has been found repeatedly that subjects tend to choose P&Q (e.g., Chicago, car); they very rarely choose ~Q. (plane). This is true especially on abstract problems, unfamiliar problems, and problems that have no social content, The result is surprising, because the logically correct answer is to pick P&~Q (Chicago, plane), as only these cards can give information about whether the rule could be false. Apparently, subjects are either not treating the task as a problem in logic, or else they are making errors in their performance of logical operations.

The possibility that subjects are acting rationally, but consider things other than the logical structure of the task to be important and relevant, is supported by a curious finding: with certain content, problems on the WST yield a very high number of logically correct (P&~Q) responses. Consider one such example (Griggs and Cox 1982):

Conditional: 'If you are in a bar drinking beer, then you must be over 19 years old."

Here are four cards that stand for four people in a bar. On one side of a card, it says what the person is drinking; on the other side it gives their age. You are a policeman checking on these four people.

Drinking Beer	16	Drinking Coke	21

Which cards would you turn over to see if anyone might be breaking the law? With this content and context, subjects usually choose the person drinking beer, and the one that is under the age of 19 (P&~Q), which is the logically correct choice. This so-called "content effect" has been observed for a variety of contents. Typically, conditionals about social rules, threats, and promises all show a facilitation in the proportion of P&~Q choices, especially if the content is familiar.

How can we explain these results? Four theories stand out in the recent literature: mental models (Johnson-Laird and Byrne 1991), heuristic-analytic theory (Evans 1989), pragmatic reasoning schemas (Cheng and Holyoak 1985; Cheng and Holyoak 1989), and social contract theory (Cosmides and Tooby 1992; Gigerenzer and Hug 1992). Johnson-Laird and Byrne's theory of mental models is one of the most comprehensive theories. It proposes that subjects construct something like a truth-table in their minds, although they do not usually make an exhaustive search of all possibilities. Subjects model the possibilities suggested by the conditional statement, by using both imagery and language. The relevance of models suggested by the context of the conditional, and the degree to which models are fleshed-out on the basis of attention to a certain model and previous experience with the situations, all determine the final picture subjects have in their minds of the possible situations that the conditional suggests. Similiar ideas are voiced by Evans (Evans 1989; Evans et al. 1993), who stressed that subjects may not be trying to solve a logical task, but rather to achieve a certain goal. According to Evans, the choices on the Wason selection task may reflect the relevance of the cards to subjects, rather than subsequent analysis of the logical structure of the problem. Other theories put emphasis on previously acquired knowledge. Cheng and Holyoak's theory of pragmatic reasoning schemas supposes that subjects use schemas (dynamic knowledge structures) whose content is in the form of general, but domain-specific rules that have been abstracted from previous experience in similar situations. Cosmides' social contract theory is perhaps the most specific theory of all, arguing that evolution has selected modular processes for reasoning about social exchange. The facilitation shown in the above example of the WST can be explained by each of these theories: subjects are led to construct more explicit models for those possibilites towards which their attention is directed; they are cued by linguistic or content effects towards choosing the most relevant cards; they possess schemas for what is socially permissible; or they possess rules for detecting cheaters on social contracts.

Although there is debate between all the theories mentioned, they have in common the notion that familiarity and social context tend to promote a mode of reasoning in which prior experience with similar situations is used to decide in the task (Note 2). All this is quite consonant with our somatic marker hypothesis, which acknowledges the same things within a more neural framework. Our psychophysiological findings (see above) showed that VM frontal damage results in decreased autonomic responsiveness 1) to stimuli with emotional meaning, and 2) to the deliberation of choices in situations in which previous experience can be used to predict outcome possibilities. Based on these findings, and on the observation that VM frontal subjects are most defective in the social domain in real life, we carried out the Wason selection task to test two hypotheses. Subjects with damage to the VM frontal cortex should differ from controls 1) in reasoning about scenarios that are familiar (have been experienced before); and 2) in reasoning about those scenarios that have the most social content.

We redesigned the WST to cast it in a more concrete mode, and to adapt it for use with brain-damaged patients. As mentioned above, we were interested not in the logical competence of subjects, but rather in comparing the reasoning of our target group of VM frontal subjects to the normal reasoning of controls. Consequently, all our stories in the WST used concrete scenarios that subjects understood and which were designed to be ecologically valid. Rather than mapping these stories onto problems in formal logic, our aim was to map them onto scenarios of reasoning of the sort that subjects would encounter in the real world, where we knew that VM frontal subjects were defective. Subjects were read stories that provided context to each conditional rule, and they had to be able to recite the story and rule from memory (this controlled for subjects who failed the task simply because they did not pay attention or could not remember the conditional rule). Cards stood for concrete objects, such as people or days of the week, and subjects were instructed to decide which of these cards they would check (turn over) if they were in the situation of the story. Cards were presented one at a time, the task and rule were reiterated each time, and the subjects had unlimited time to make their decisions. After all cards had been presented, they were left in front of the subject, and an opportunity was provided for the subjects to change their minds, on any of the choices. The final choice that subjects said they were happy with was the one recorded. All subjects were selected from our patient registry and had been fully characterized neuroanatomically and neuropsychologically as part of an ongoing program project (Damasio and Damasio 1989). Three groups of subjects were used: patients with damage centered on the VM frontal cortex, patients with damage centered on the DL frontal cortex (specifically excluding the VM cortex), and patients with damage outside the frontal cortex. Subjects were chosen such that all three groups were matched on verbal and performance IQ (ca. 100 ± 12 for all groups). All three groups were also similar in age and educational background. All VM frontal subjects, and most other subjects, repeated the experiment at least once, typically on separate visits to our clinic. The neuroanatomy for our VM frontal subjects is shown in Figure 3. We present data here only from that subset of stories for which reproducible responses within subject groups were obtained.

Experiment 1: Patients with VM Frontal Lesions Are Impaired on Reasoning in Familiar Domains

We hypothesized that patients with VM frontal lesions would be impaired (differ from controls) on reasoning in those domains that especially utilize somatic markers. One factor in the extent to which these markers are used may be the familiarity of the situation: reasoning in familiar domains could make use of previous experience via the mechanism of somatic markers. We used three groups of subjects: six with VM frontal lesions (one subject of seven never chose any cards at all. As we were interested in more specific effects in this experiment, we excluded this subject here), seven with DL frontal lesions, and 23 with lesions elsewhere. We presented subjects with two concrete scenarios, neither of which involved a social contract. The two stories differed in the amount of familiarity subjects presumably had with them. The conditional rules were:

(a) less familiar: "If you eat the chili, then you will order a beer"
(b) more familiar: "When it's humid and muggy, it will rain in the afternoon"

Several subjects had not ever eaten chili, and although the rule made sense, few subjects would have actually experienced it in action (at least in the Midwest) or ever been engaged in deciding if the rule is true or false on past occasions. Most subjects agreed with the weather rule, and many subjects who were farmers further elaborated on details. Nearly all subjects from the Midwest should have experienced this rule in action many times throughout the summer months, and would have been interested in deciding on its validity on past occasions. Consistent with the literature of reasoning on non-social stories such as these, both these stories tended to elicit P&Q as the most frequent response from controls. Subjects were apparently interested more in finding confirming instances than in finding an exception to the rule.

Subjects tended to choose slightly more P&Q cards on the weather rule, and found it easier than the chili rule. VM frontal subjects showed no such tendency: the proportion of P&Q cards they chose varied negatively with familiarity of the story context (Fig. 4). Thus, although some VM frontal subjects chose P&Q on the unfamiliar story, as did controls, none of the VM frontal subjects chose this card

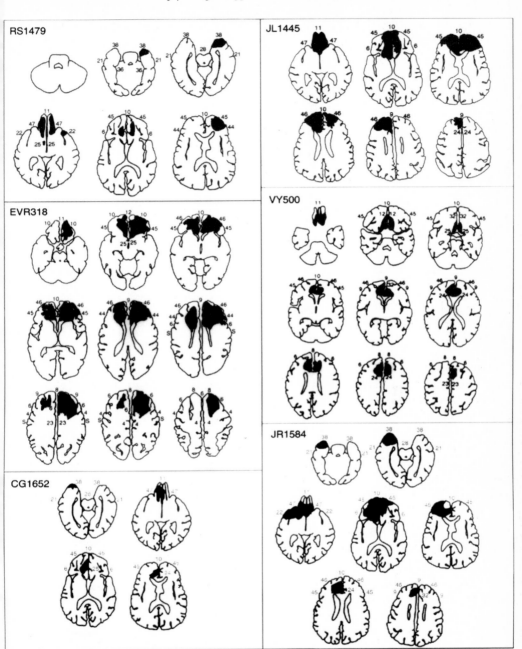

Fig. 3. Templates of sites of lesions for the six VM frontal subjects used in the Wason selection task experiments. Dark regions correspond to lesioned tissue. All templates were prepared according to our standard methods (Damasio and Damasio 1989), from MRI or CT scans of the subjects' brains

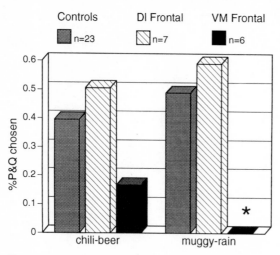

Fig. 4. Percent of P&Q card choices on reasoning about stories that did not involve social contracts. Subjects were read stories and provided with two conditional rules: "If you eat chili then you will order a beer," and "If it is a humid and muggy day, then it will rain in the afternoon." The most common response choice for both stories from the controls was P&Q. VM frontal subjects differed significantly from both brain-damaged controls and from DL frontal subjects on the weather rule

combination on the more familiar story. A chi-square test of the frequencies with which different subject groups endorsed certain card choices was significant only for frequencies of P&Q on the more familiar story (chi-square = 8.3; p = 0.016). An examination of the residuals revealed that it was the VM frontal subjects that differed from the other two groups. We consequently pooled the control and DL frontal groups. When this pooled group was compared to the VM frontal group, a significantly different frequency of choosing P&Q on the weather rule was seen (p = 0.006; Fisher's exact test).

These results are consistent with the hypothesis that subjects use memory of previously encountered similar circumstances when reasoning on familiar problems. Lesions of the VM frontal cortex appear to impair this contributory mechanism of reasoning.

Experiment 2: Subjects with VM Frontal Lesions Are Most Impaired in Reasoning on Familiar Social Problems

The most severe impairments following VM frontal damage are evident in the social domain in the real world. Our initial hypothesis (hypothesis #2 above) was that VM frontal subjects would differ most from controls on the WST when confronted with social stories. However, our findings below suggest that the effect is more specific than that: subjects with VM frontal lesions differ only on those social stories that are most familiar.

We used the same three subject groups as in Experiment 1. Three stories within the context of a social contract were presented: in each story, subjects were told to check for people who might be cheating on a rule. The conditionals were:

(a) less familiar: "If you work on a weekend, then you get a day off during the week."
(b) less familiar: "If you get a pension, then you must have worked for the company for at least 10 years."
(c) more familiar: "If you are drinking beer, you must be under the age of 19."

Although all three stories were concrete and made sense, stories (a) and (b) would not be likely to have been actually encountered by subjects. In each of these two stories, subjects were cued into the perspective of a suspicious employee who thinks the company he is working for may be cheating on the rule that they have promised their employees. (We also used the same stories with the roles reversed, i.e., subjects were the employer instead of the employee, and found similar results). It is unlikely that any subject would have ever had occasion to test either of these particular rules. Story (c), however, would be a rule that subjects had probably actually had experience with and would have probably examined for violations on previous occasions. All subjects (including the VM frontal subjects) said they found story (c) easier than the other two stories.

Figure 5 shows the results from our experiment. Subjects tended to choose P&~Q on these tasks, as has been reported in the literature. Groups did not differ significantly in their endorsement of P&~Q on the two unfamiliar stories, although the DL frontal subjects appeared to perform slightly differently from the other

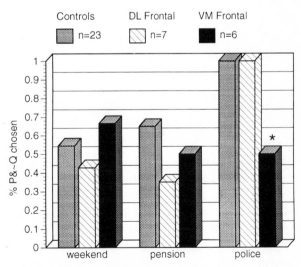

Fig. 5. Percent of P&~Q card choices on reasoning about social rules. Subjects were provided with three conditional rules: "If you work on the weekend, then you get a day off during the week," "If you get a pension, then you must have worked for the company for at least 10 years," "If you are drinking beer, you must be under the age of 19." The most common response choice was P&~Q. Subjects with VM frontal lesions differed significantly from the other groups only on the beer drinking story

groups, perhaps as a result of the complexity of the problem. However, on the familiar social story, every single control and every single DL frontal subject chose P&~Q; all found the task very easy. Dramatically, the VM frontal subjects did not show this facilitation when the subject matter was familiar. Groups differed on the familiar story in the frequency with which they chose P&~Q (chi-square = 8.4; p = 0.015) and unusual card combinations (chi-square = 13, p = 0.0015). Since the controls and DL frontals performed identically, their results were pooled; comparisons between the pooled group and the VM frontal group showed a significant effect of group on the frequency with which P&~Q was chosen on the beer-drinking rule (p = 0.03; Fisher's exact test).

Interestingly, the facilitation of the P&~Q response between non-social and social-contract stories was present for all subject groups. Counter to our original hypothesis, VM frontal subjects were normal in choosing more P&~Q combinations on stories involving social contracts (chi-square test: p > 0.1), but they did not show any facilitation when the material was made more familiar. We computed all response combinations that subjects gave (all combinations of the four cards chosen) on all different stories, four of which are shown in Figure 6. It was only on familiar stories, both social and non-social, that the VM frontal group differed significantly from the other two groups. On familiar non-social stories, the VM frontal subjects chose fewer P&Q cards (the most common response on non-social stories) than the other two groups. On familiar social-contract stories, the VM frontal subjects chose fewer P&~Q cards (the most common response on social stories) than the other two groups (who chose 100% P&~Q). Thus, subjects with VM frontal lesions fail to reason normally about familiar scenarios, both social and non-social (Fig. 7).

The VM frontal subjects had a larger variance in their responses as a group than did the other groups. We considered the possibility that their responses were simply noisier, or more random, and that this could account for the data. Since each subject had repeated the task on separate days, we simply compared performance on the two trials. We found that VM frontal subjects were as consistent in their choices as subjects in the other groups. Random or inconsistent behavior cannot account for our results. There was, however, a general tendency by the VM frontal subjects to choose fewer cards, as reported in the next section.

Experiment 3: Patients with Lesions of the VM Frontal Cortex Check Fewer Situations than Controls Do

Our somatic marker hypothesis led us to predict that subjects with damage to the VM frontal cortex would tend to check fewer cards than control subjects. Our reasoning was that subjects with VM frontal cortex lesions would not engage somatic markers, and would therefore not be prompted to check situations that would normally be linked to a somatic marker.

We presented six stories to our three subject groups. The WST was administered on each of these six stories according to our modified paradigm. We re-

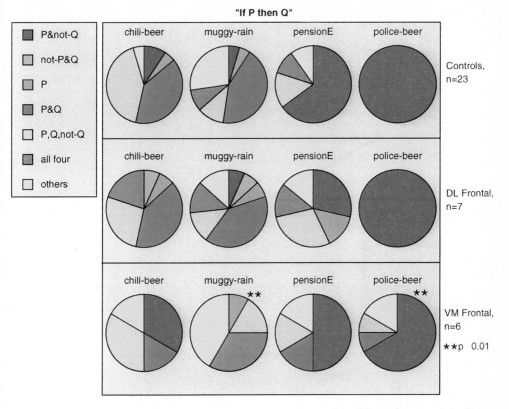

Fig. 6. Summary of response choices for the three subject groups on four of the stories we used. Card combinations chosen are indicated by color, and the proportion of the combination that was chosen is indicated by its area in the pie graph. Each row represents the choices made by one of the three subject groups, and each pie stands for a different story. Not all stories and not all card combinations are shown here. We examined the frequencies of all possible card combinations on all the stories and only found two cases where frequencies differed significantly between groups (chi-square test with subsequent Fisher exact test). These corresponded to the most common combinations on the most familiar stories (P&Q for the muggy-rain rule, and P&~Q) for the police-beer rule)

corded the total number of cards that subjects decided to check for each story. Control subjects and subjects with dorsolateral frontal lesions did not differ on this variable and their data were pooled.

Figure 8 shows the mean numbers of cards (minimum = 0, maximum = 4) that subjects in each group picked. There was no effect of the type of story, and we show the mean for all six stories. Subjects with VM frontal lesions (n = 7) tended to choose fewer cards on all stories than did controls (n = 22). This effect was significant despite a large variance in the VM group (two-sample t-test for unequal variances: $t[8] = -10.1$; $p < 0.0001$). Some subjects in the VM group did not choose any cards at all for a story, and one subject chose no cards for any of the six stories, something no control did (this subject had been excluded from Experiments 1 and 2 above).

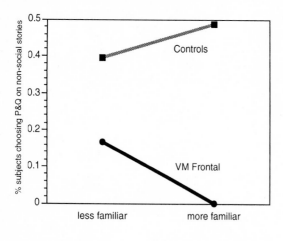

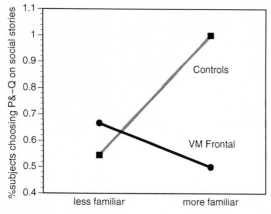

Fig. 7. Subjects with VM frontal lesions reason abnormally on scenarios that are most familiar. At the top, proportion of most common response on non social stories; at the bottom, proportion of most common response in stories involving social contracts. In each case, subjects with VM frontal lesions differ most from controls (brain-damaged controls and DL frontal subjects pooled) on the more familiar story. Whereas controls show a facilitation of the response combination when the story is more familiar, subjects with VM frontal lesions show no such facilitation, or even do worse. The results support the hypothesis that lesions of the VM frontal cortex impair the ability to deploy reasoning mechanisms that make use of prior experience in familiar situations

We followed up these results with a case study, K.C., who showed just the opposite trend from the VM frontal subjects (Fig. 8). K.C. had a medial prefrontal cyst, which resulted in epileptic activity. It is thus likely that his VM frontal cortex was more active, at least at times, than that of controls. K.C. tended to pick many, often all, cards for each story. Worried that he might have missed something, he checked all possibilities, whereas patients with lesions in the same brain region tended to check none. We thus have the observation that decrease or increase of activity in the VM frontal cortex appears to correlate with a decrease or increase, respectively, in the number of choices that are examined as important for the subject. While these data will need to be corroborated with explicitly designed

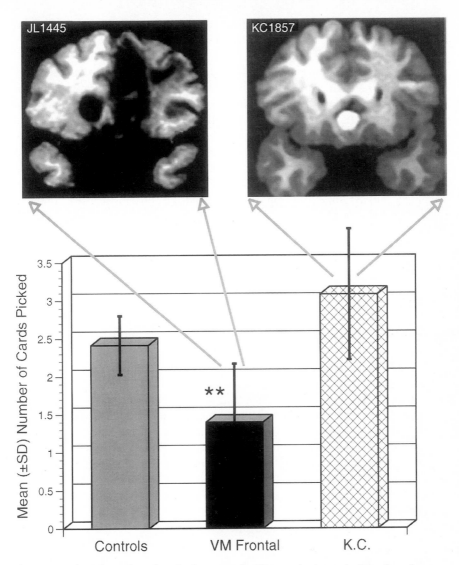

Fig. 8. Mean (± SD) number of cards chosen on the Wason selection task. Bars show the mean performance on 6 different stories. Subjects with VM frontal lesions chose significantly fewer cards than did controls (brain-damaged controls and DL frontal subjects pooled). A converse example was provided by patient K.C., who had epileptic activity in the frontal cortex due to a mesial frontal cyst. MRI scans of K.C. (right) and a representative VM frontal subject (left) are shown at the very top of the figure: whereas VM frontal subjects have lesions of the VM frontal cortex, K.C.'s VM frontal cortex was intact and probably abnormally hyperactive due to irritation by his cyst (white circular object in scan)

studies, they are very consistent with the predictions that the somatic marker hypothesis makes.

It is interesting to note that these findings are consistent with the picture of prefrontal activity that has been gleaned from patients with obsessive-compulsive disorder. Such patients suffer from the urge to check and worry about possibilities that people normally ignore. PET imaging has shown that the symptoms of obsessive-compulsive disorder correlate with increased activity in the VM frontal cortex (Baxter et al. 1988; Rauch et al. 1994).

Our findings are consonant with a hypothesized role of the VM frontal cortex in mediating the elicitation of emotional states that serve to direct attention towards stimuli and that serve to guide behavior on the basis of the emotional valence aroused. In control subjects, this directs their attention to some of the cards and prompts them to investigate what might be on the other side of the card. Ventromedial frontal patients, on the other hand, are not attentionally directed and are not prompted: their interest is not aroused. K.C. provides the reverse picture: he worries obsessively whether he should check more cards, just in case he might have missed something important, and ends up choosing nearly all of them.

Discussion

The discussion below focuses on the Wason Selection Task studies that we just described.

Synopsis of Findings

We found that subjects with VM frontal lesions 1) tended to choose fewer cards, 2) differed from controls in their choice of particular card combinations only on those stories that were most familiar, and 3) showed no facilitation of logically correct responses on social stories with increasing familiarity. These findings suggest a revision of our original hypothesis that lesions of the VM frontal cortex specifically impair reasoning in the social domain. Rather, it appears to be reasoning in familiar domains, social or not, that is most impaired with VM frontal lesions. Possibly, reasoning in social contexts draws heavily upon prior experience, and that may be why social behavior is especially impaired in this patient population.

Theories of Reasoning

What might be special about reasoning in familiar social domains? One important difference concerns the speed with which one needs to make a decision. If you are deciding what to investigate in a non-social situation, you have more time to make your choice, and you can afford to examine confirming rather than disconfirming instances. However, if you are the policeman checking for someone breaking the law, the situation is more dynamic: as soon as the cheaters see you checking for them, they will try to evade you. It is this reciprocity in social situations that calls for a premium on speed and on attention to disconfirming instances of the rule. Such pressures during evolution may have resulted in a system designed to use previous knowledge, in the form of rapid, somatic signalling.

The reason for the different performance of VM frontal subjects on familiar non-social stories is more complicated to explain, since the most common response from the controls (P&Q) is not the logically correct response in the first place. As we pointed out earlier, this response may, however, be quite rational in light of what it is that subjects are interested in. In the case of the weather rule, for example, a high proportion of P&Q seems rational if one assumes that it is potentially dangerous/negative outcomes that interest the subjects: they want to see if it is raining when it is muggy. The possibility of sunshine is not an interesting exploration, since it is a harmless outcome. Although this issue will need more experimental attention to be sorted out, we suggest that a similar mechanism may operate in familiar social and familiar non-social situations. When the situation is unfamiliar, subjects rely more on propositional and content-insensitive reasoning strategies. When the situation is familiar, an additional mechanism is employed: reasoning by analogy to previous experience. An important component (though by no means all) of this reasoning-by-analogy makes use of non-propositional (overt and covert) neural processes: specifically, the elicitation of a feeling that is based on previous experience with similar situations. We propose that what VM frontal subjects lack is the device by which they can trigger such feelings. A similar function for the VM frontal cortex in generating "feelings of familiarity" has been proposed by Pribram (Pribram 1987), on the basis of primate experiments.

Comparison to Other Models

Our results and theory find resonance in several other recent psychological theories of how emotion and reason might be related. Two theories in particular that are worth discussing are Shallice's (Shallice and Burgess 1991, 1993) proposal that a supervisory system of decision-making resides in the frontal lobes, and Zajonc's (Zajonc 1980; Zajonc and Kunst-Wilson 1980) writings on the primacy of affect in choice.

Shallice and Burgess (Shallice and Burgess 1991, 1993) have elaborated an earlier information-processing model (Norman and Shallice 1986). In their scheme, there are two basic modes of reasoning: routine operations rely on an automatic device for allocating resources to one of many decision-making schemas; novel situations, however, must invoke a supervisory system that activates schemas via non-routine mechanisms. The neural substrate of the supervisory system is postulated to reside in the frontal lobes. An important component of Shallice's model is markers that serve to interrupt ongoing behavior and redirect the flow of control in the decision-making system. No anatomical basis for these markers has been made explicit, but their function is certainly analogous to the somatic markers in our theory.

A second important theory for comparison originates in the work of Robert Zajonc. Building on the finding that people prefer those stimuli they have encountered most frequently (Zajonc 1968), Zajonc carried out experiments in which subjects were exposed to subliminal stimuli. Although subjects were unable to recognize the stimuli subsequently, they exhibited preferences for those stimuli to which they were exposed most frequently (Zajonc and Kunst-Wilson 1980). On the basis of these results, Zajonc argued that "preferences need no inferences", i.e., that emotional processes were prior to, and faster than, cognitive and inferential processes. The recent literature suggests a somewhat modified view: subliminal exposure results in implicit memory of the stimuli, rendering them more distinct (Mandler et al. 1987), easier to process (Bornstein 1992), and capable of eliciting a feeling of familiarity when encountered again (Bonanno and Stillings 1986). Other recent findings support these views. Implicit memory for previously encountered events can be recalled in the form of a feeling about that event, and such feelings serve to focus attention and bias choices when judgments have to be made (Klinger and Greenwald 1994). We find this framework congenial. An important role must be assigned to memory for past events that is implicit and that can guide behavior in the form of a feeling. We suggest that somatic markers are precisely such a mechanism (Note 3).

In conclusion, we have shown that lesions of the VM frontal cortex impair the ability to give normal autonomic responses to emotionally significant stimuli, and to the process of deliberating decisions on a gambling task, and that they also impair the ability to reason normally in familiar domains. Our proposal is that these two findings are two sides of the same coin: the VM frontal cortex engages reasoning mechanisms in familiar domains that require the evocation of somatic states.

The idea that human behavior is generated by domain-insensitive, general processes as well as by context-dependent and emotional ones is not entirely new. Aristotle suggested a similar possibility when he made a distinction between reason and passion. What is new is the idea that "reason" in fact subsumes both processes and is not allied only with the first one. Also new is the hypothesis that context-dependent reasoning relies on feeling, and that feeling is body-based. These suggestions run counter to viewpoints that have become heavily entrenched in modern cognitive science, and that are probably best characterized as Neo-Cartesian (Damasio 1994).

Notes

Note 1. This is only true loosely speaking, of course. The situation is complicated by the fact that adaptation in an evolutionary context needs to refer not to the individual's fitness but to inclusive fitness. Excepting phenomena such as altruism, what is good for an individual will also generally be good in terms of inclusive fitness. We are making the assumption that, for our subjects, their reasoning was rational insofar as their goal was to achieve adaptive solutions to problems. But their goals may not always have been the goal of giving the logically correct answer to a problem, contrary to the goal as judged in the eyes of the experimenter.

Note 2. This claim is consistent with Cosmides' (Cosmides 1989; Cosmides and Tooby 1992) hypothesis that there are innate mechanisms for reasoning about social exchange, but includes the modification that innate mechanisms can only pre-set certain parameters and cannot account for all performance. Innate mechanisms that have been sculpted by evolution can be such that they in turn predispose the organism to learn about social encounters in a particular way. The ability to reason in familiar social domains is then the result of both innate and learned knowledge working together.

Note 3. Implicit memory has diverse substrates. Our experiments have tested one particular substrate, autonomic response. There are many other routes that are all likely to play a role in guiding choice by prior experience. In addition to the projections from the VM prefrontal cortex to the amygdala and to autonomic control nuclei, these will include projections to neuromodulatory brainstem nuclei and the basal forebrain. Our proposal is that the function of an implicit or explicit memory in guiding decision-making will depend specifically on a memory of what happened to the organism previously, i.e., how the body felt at that time. Thus, somatic markers always use either representations of previous body state, or an actual somatic state, but in each case the topic of the marker is the relation between the outcome of a prior decision and its effect on the body.

Acknowledgments. We thank Charles Rockland for helpful discussion. This study was supported by NINDS grant NS 19632. R.A. is a Burroughs-Wellcome Fund Fellow of the Life Sciences Research Foundation.

References

Barbas H, Henion THH, Dermon CR (1991) Diverse thalamic projections to the prefrontal cortex in the rhesus monkey. J Comp Neurol 313:65–94

Baxter LR, Schwartz JM, Mazziotta JC, Phelps ME, Pahl JJ, Guze BH, Fairbanks L (1988) Cerebral glucose metabolic rates in nondepressed patients with obsessive-compulsive disorder. Am J Psychiat 145:1560–1563

Bechara A, Damasio AR, Damasio H, Anderson SW (1994) Insensitivity to future consequences following damage to human prefrontal cortex. Cognition 50:7–15

Bechara A, Tranel D, Damasio H, Damasio AR (in press) Failure to respond autonomically to anticipated future outcomes following damage to prefrontal cortex. Cerebral Cortex (in press)

Bonanno GA, Stillings NA (1986) Preference, familiarity and recognition after repeated brief exposures to random geometric shapes. Am J Psychol 99:403–415

Bornstein RF (1992) Subliminal mere exposure effects. In: Bornstein RF, Pittman TS (eds) Perception without awareness. New York, Guilford Press, pp 191–210

Carroll JB (1993) Human cognitive abilities: a survey of factor-analytic studies. New York, Cambridge University Press

Cheng PW, Holyoak KJ (1985) Pragmatic reasoning schemas. Cog Psychol 17:391–416

Cheng PW, Holyoak KJ (1989) On the natural selection of reasoning theories. Cognition 33:285–313

Cosmides L (1989) The logic of social exchange: has natural selection shaped how humans reason? Studies with the Wason selection task. Cognition 31:187–276

Cosmides L, Tooby J (1992) Cognitive adaptations for social exchange. In: Barkow JH, Cosmides L, Tooby J (eds) The adapted mind: evolutionary psychology and the generation of culture New York, Oxford University Press, pp 163–228

Damasio AR (1994) Descartes' Error: Emotion, Reason, and the Human Brain. New York: Grosset/ Putnam (Published in France and England by Editions Odile Jacob, Paris (1995), and by Picador/ MacMillan, London (1995))

Damasio AR (1995) Toward a neurobiology of emotion and feeling: operational concepts and hypotheses. The Neuroscientist 1:19–25

Damasio H, Damasio AR (1989) Lesion analysis in neuropsychology. New York, Oxford University Press

Damasio AR, Tranel D, Damasio H (1990) Individuals with sociopathic behavior caused by frontal damage fail to respond autonomically to social stimuli. Behav Brain Res 41:81–94

Damasio AR, Tranel D, Damasio H (1991) Somatic markers and the guidance of behavior: Theory and preliminary testing. In: Levin HS, Eisenberg HM, Benton AL (eds) Frontal lobe function and dysfunction. New York, Oxford University Press, pp 217–229

Damasio H, Grabowski T, Frank R, Galburda AM, Damasio AR (1994) The return of Phineas Gage: Clues about the brain from the skull of a famous patient. Science 264:1102–1104

Diamond A, Goldman-Rakic PS (1989) Comparison of human infants and rhesus monkeys on Piaget's A-not B task: evidence for dependence on dorsolateral prefrontal cortex. Exp Brain Res 74:24–40

Ebbeson EB, Konecni VJ (1980) On the external validity of decision-making research: What do we know about decisions in the real world? In: Wallsten TS (eds) Cognitive processes in choice and decision behavior. Hillsdale, NJ, Lawrence Erlbaum Associates, pp 128–144

Eslinger PJ, Damasio AR (1985) Severe disturbance of higher cognition after bilateral frontal lobe ablation: patient EVR. Neurology 35:1731–1741

Evans JSt BT (1989) Bias in Human Reasoning: Causes and Consequences, Hove, UK, Lawrence Erlbaum Associates

Evans JSt BT (1993) Bias and rationality. In: Manktelow KI, Over DE (eds) Rationality, London, Routledge

Evans JSt BT, Newstead SE, Byrne RMJ (1993) Human reasoning: the psychology of deduction. Hillsdale (USA): Lawrence Erlbaum Associates

Fodor JA (1983) The Modularity of Mind. MIT Press

Funahashi S, Chafee MV, Goldman-Rakic PS (1993) Prefrontal neuronal activity in rhesus monkeys performing a delayed anti-saccade task. Nature 365:753–756

Fuster JM (1989) The prefrontal cortex. Anatomy, physiology, and neuropsychology of the frontal lobe. New York, Raven Press

Gigerenzer G, Hug K (1992) Domain-specific reasoning: social contracts, cheating, and perspective change. Cognition 43:127–171

Goldman-Rakic PS (1988) Topography of cognition: parallel distributed networks in primate association cortex. Ann Rev Neurosci 11:137–156

Goldman-Rakic PS (1990) Cellular and circuit basis of working memory in prefrontal cortex of nonhuman primates. Prog Brain Res 85:325–336

Griggs RA, Cox JR (1982) The elusive thematic-materials effect in Wason's selection task. Brit J Psychol 73:407–420

Johnson-Laird PN, Byrne RMJ (1991) Deduction. Hove (UK): Lawrence Erlbaum Associates

Klinger MR, Greenwald AG (1994) Preferences need no inferences? The cognitive basis of unconscious mere exposure effects. In: Niedenthal PM, Kitayama S (eds) The heart's eye: emotional influences in perception and attention. New York: Academic Press, pp 68–86

Kowalska DM, Bachevalier J, Mishkin M (1991) The role of the inferior prefrontal convexity in performance of delayed nonmatching-to-sample. Neuropsychologia 29:583–600

Levin HS, Eisenberg HM, Benton AL (1991) Frontal lobe function and dysfunction. New York, Oxford University Press

Mandler G, Nakamura Y, Van Zandt BJS (1987) Nonspecific effects of exposure to stimuli that cannot be recognized. J Exp Psychol 13:646–648

Manktelow KL, Over DE (1987) Reasoning and rationality. Mind Language 2:199–219

Morecraft RJ, Geula C, Mesulam M-M (1992) Cytoarchitecture and neural afferents of orbitofrontal cortex in the brain of the monkey. J Comp Neurol 323:341–358

Norman DA, Shallice T (1986) Attention to action: willed and automatic control of behavior. In: Davidson RJ, Schwartz GE, Shapiro D (eds) Consciousness and self-regulation. New York, Plenum, pp 1–18

Pandya DN, Barnes CL (1987) Architecture and connections of the frontal lobe. In: Perecman E (ed) The Frontal lobes revisited. New York, IRBN Press, pp 41–68

Passingham RE (1972) Visual discrimination learning after selective prefrontal cortical ablations in monkeys (Macaca mulatta). Neuropsychologia 10:27–39

Pribram KH (1987) The subdivisions of the frontal cortex revisited. In: Perecman E (ed) The Frontal lobes revisited. New York, IRBN Press, pp 11–34

Rauch SL, Jenike MA, Alpert NM, Baer L, Breiter HCR, Savage CR, Fischman AJ (1994) Regional cerebral blood flow measured during symptom provocation in obsessive-compulsive disorder using oxygen 15-labelled carbon dioxide and positron emission tomography. Arch Gen Psychiat 51:62–70

Rips LJ (1983) Cognitive processes in propositional reasoning. Psychol Rev 90:38–71

Rosenkilde CE (1979) Functional heterogeneity of the prefrontal cortex. Behav Neural Biol 25:301–345

Shallice T, Burgess P (1991) Higher-order cognitive impairments and frontal lobe lesions in man. In: Levin HS, Eisenberg HM, Benton AL (eds) Frontal lobe function and dysfunction. New York, Oxford University Press, pp 125–138

Shallice T, Burgess P (1993) Supervisory control of action and thought selection. In: Baddeley A, Weiskrantz L (eds) Attention: selection, awareness, and control. Oxford, UK, Clarendon Press, pp 171–187

Stich SP (1985) Could man be an irrational animal? Synthese 64:115–135

Sutherland S (1992) Irrationality: the enemy within. London, Constable

Tranel D (1994) "Acquired sociopathy:" The development of sociopathic behavior following focal brain damage. In: Fowles DC (ed) Progress in experimental personality and psychopathology research. New York, Springer Publishing Co, pp 285–312

Tranel D, Damasio H (1994) Neuroanatomical correlates of electrodermal skin conductance responses. Psychophysiology 31:427–438

Voytko ML (1985) Cooling orbital frontal cortex disrupts matching-to-sample and visual discrimination learning in monkeys. Physiol Psychol 13:219–229

Wason PC (1966) Reasoning. In: Foss BM (ed) New horizons in psychology. Harmondsworth: Penguin, pp 135–151

Wason PC, Johnson-Laird PN (1972) Psychology of reasoning: structure and content. London, Batsford

Wason PC, Shapiro D (1971) Natural and contrived experience in a reasoning problem. Quart J Exp Psychol 23:63–71

Wilson FAW, Scalaidhe SPO, Goldman-Rakic PS (1993) Dissociation of object and spatial processing domains in primate prefrontal cortex. Science 260:1955–1958

Zajonc RB (1968) Attitudinal effects of mere exposure. J Personality Social Psychol Mon 9:1–27

Zajonc RB (1980) Feeling and thinking: preferences need no inferences. Am Psychol 35:151–175

Zajonc RB, Kunst-Wilson WR (1980) Affective discrimination of stimuli that cannot be recognized. Science 207:557–558

Feeling Reasons

P.S. Churchland

Introduction: The Social Significance of Agent Autonomy and Responsibility

Much of human social life depends on the notion that agents have control over their actions and are responsible for their choices. We assume that it is sensible to punish and reward behavior so long as the person was in control and chose knowingly and intentionally. Without the assumptions of agent control and responsibility, human social commerce is hardly conceivable. As members of a social species, we recognize cooperation, loyalty, and reciprocation as prominent features of the social environment, and we react with hostility when group members disappoint socially salient expectations. Inflicting disutilities on the socially renegade and rewarding civic virtue helps restore the standards. In other social species, too, social unreliability, such as failures to reciprocate grooming or food-sharing, provokes a reaction likely to cost the renegade animal or his kin, sooner or later. For example, de Waal (1982) observed that chimpanzees who renege on a supportive coalition when loyalty is needed will later suffer retaliation. In social mammals at least, mechanisms for keeping the social order seem to be part of what evolution bequeathed to brain circuitry (Clutton-Brock and Parker 1995). The stability of the social-expectation baseline is sufficiently important to survival that individuals are prepared to incur some cost in enforcing those expectations. Just as an anubis baboon learns that tasty scorpions are to be found under rocks but cannot just be picked up, so it learns that failure to reciprocate grooming when it is duly expected may yield a smart slap. Much of behavior is guided by the expectation of certain consequences – not only what will happen in the physical world, but including also what will happen in the social world (Cheney and Seyfarth 1990; de Waal 1989).

What is it – for us or baboons or chimpanzees – to have control over one's behavior? Are we really responsible for our choices and decisions? Will neuroscientific understanding of the neuronal mechanisms for decision-making change how we think about these fundamental features of social commerce? These are some of the questions I wish to consider in this essay.

Department of Philosophy, B-002, University of California, La Jolla CA 92093, USA

A.R. Damasio et al. (Eds.)
Neurobiology of Decision-Making
© Springer-Verlag Berlin Heidelberg 1996

Are We Responsible and In Control if Our Choices and Actions Are *Caused*?

A venerable tradition bases the conditions for free will and control on a contrast between being caused to do something and not being so caused. For example, if someone pushes me from behind and I bump into you, then my bumping you was caused by the push; I did not choose to bump you. Examples conforming to this prototype have given credence to the idea that in order for a choice to be free, it must be uncaused. That is, it is supposed that a free choice is made when, without prior cause and without prior constraints, a decision comes into being and an action results. This contracausal construal free choice is known as libertarianism (see Campbell 1957). Is it plausible?

As Hume pointed out in 1739,[1] the answer is surely no. Hume argued that our choices and decisions are in fact caused by other events in the mind: desires, beliefs, preferences, feelings, and so forth. Neither do the precipitating events, whether described as mental or as neuronal, need to be conscious. He also made the much deeper and more penetrating observation that agents are not considered responsible for the choices they made unless they are caused by our desires, intentions, and so forth. Randomness, pure chance, and utter unpredictability are not preconditions for control. Hume puts the issue with memorable compactness:

where [actions] proceed not from some cause in the characters and disposition of the person, who perform'd them, they infix not themselves upon him, and can neither redound to his honor if good, nor infamy, if evil. (p. 411)

Logic reveals, Hume argued, that responsibility is actually inconsistent with libertarianism (uncaused choice). Someone may choose to climb onto his roof because he does not want the rain to come in his house, he wants to fix the loose shingles, and he believes that he needs to get up on the roof to do that. His desires, intentions and beliefs are part of the causal antecedents resulting in his choice. If, without determining desire and belief, he simply went up onto the roof – as it were, for no reason – his sanity and hence his control is seriously in doubt. More generally, a choice undetermined by anything the agent believes, intends or desires is actually the kind of thing we consider out of the agent's control and not the sort of thing for which we hold someone responsible. Furthermore, desires or beliefs, were *they* uncaused rather than caused by other stable features of the person's character and temperament, are likewise inappropriate preconditions for responsible choice (see also Hobart 1934).

Neither Hume's argument that choices are internally caused nor his argument showing that libertarianism is absurd has even been convincingly refuted (for disagreements with Hume, see Kenny 1989). Notice, moreover, that his arguments hold whether or not one thinks of the mind as a separate Cartesian substance or as a pattern of activity of the physical brain; whether one thinks of the etiologically

---

[1] In his anonymously published, *A Treatise on Human Nature*. Edited by LA Selby-Bigge (first printing 1888).

relevant states as conscious or unconscious. If anything in philosophy could count as a result. Hume's argument on free will does. Nonetheless, the idea that randomness in the physical world is somehow the key to what makes free choice free remains appealing to those inclined to believe that free choice must be uncaused choice. The appeal of quantum mechanics, chaos, and so forth as a "solution" to the problem of free will and responsibility generally derives from an intuition innocent of exposure to Hume's result.

If all behavior is caused, what is the difference between voluntary and involuntary actions? When, if ever, is an agent responsible? Many possibilities have been explored in attempts to explain how the notions of control and responsibility can make sense in the context of causation, of determinism. To begin with, it is clear that the distinction between internal and external causes will not suffice to distinguish the voluntary from the involuntary. A patient with Huntington's disease cannot prevent himself from making choreoform movements; a sleepwalker may unplug the phone or kick the dog; a phobic patient may have an overwhelming urge to wash her hands. The cause of the behavior in each of these cases is internal, in the subject's brain. Yet the behavior is considered to be out of the agent's control.

Another strategy is to base the distinction on felt differences in inner experience between those actions we choose to do and those over which we feel we have no control. Thus it allegedly feels different when we evince a cry as a startle response to a mouse leaping out of the compost heap, and when we cry out to get someone's attention. Is introspection a reliable guide to responsibility? Can introspection distinguish those internal causes for which we are responsible from those for which we are not? (see also Crick 1994). Probably not. There are undoubtedly many cases where introspection is no guide at all. Phobic patients, obsessive-compulsive patients, and Touretters are obvious examples that muddy the waters. The various kinds of addictions present further difficulties. A contented smoker typically feels that the desire for a cigarette is indeed his, and that his reaching for a cigarette feels as free as reaching to turn on the television. Not so the smoker who is trying to quit the habit. The increase in intensity of sexual interest and desire at puberty is surely the result of hormonal changes on the brain, not something over which one has much control. Yet engaging in certain activities, such as ogling the opposite sex, feels as free as tying one's shoes. More problematic perhaps are the many examples from everyday life where one may suppose the decision was entirely one's own, only to discover that subtle manipulation of desires had in fact been the decisive factor. According to the fashion standards of the day, one finds certain clothes beautiful, others frumpy, and the choice of wardrobe seems, introspectively, as free as any choice. There is no escaping, however, the fact that what is in fashion has a huge effect on what we find beautiful in clothes, and this affects not only choice in clothes, but also such things as aesthetic judgment regarding plumpness or slenderness of the female body.

Social psychologists have produced dozens of examples that further muddy the waters, but a simple one will convey the point. On a table in a shopping mall, experimenters placed ten pairs of identical panty hose, and asked shoppers to select a pair, and then briefly explain their choice. After selection, the choosers referred to color, denier, sheerness and so forth, as their rationale. In fact, there was a huge position effect: shoppers tended to pick the pantyhose in the rightmost position on the table and, in fact, the panty hose were identical and differed not at all in color, sheerness and so on. None of the subjects considered position to be a factor; none of them referred to it as a basis for choice, yet it clearly was so. Other examples of priming, subliminal perception, emotional manipulation, etc., make introspection a highly unreliable guide.

In a different attack on the problem, philosophers have explored the idea that if the choice was free, the agent could have chosen otherwise, that in some sense, the agent had the power to do something else (see Taylor 1974; Kenny 1989). The weakness in the strategy shows up when we ask further, "what exactly does that mean?" If all behavior has antecedent causes, then "could have done otherwise" seems to boil down to "would have done otherwise if antecedent conditions had been different." Accepting that equivalence means the criterion is too weak to distinguish between the shouted insults of a Touretter, whose tics include random and undirected outbursts ("idiot, idiot, idiot"), and those of a member of parliament responding to an honorable member's proposal ("idiot, idiot, idiot"). In both cases, had the antecedent conditions been different, obviously the results would have been different. Nevertheless, we hold the parliamentarian responsible, but not the Touretter.

In our legal as well as our daily practice, the pattern is to accept certain prototypical conditions as excusing a person from responsibility, but to assume him responsible unless a specific exculpatory condition obtains. In other words, responsibility is the default condition; excuse from and mitigation of responsibility has to be established. The set of conditions regarded as exculpatory can be modified as we learn more about behavior and its etiology. Thus a child Touretter might have been smacked for his ticcing outbursts in public, until it is understood that the tics are not within his control and that punishment is totally inefficacious.

Aristotle was the first to articulate this strategy, and the core of his ideas on this matter is still reflected in much of human practice, including current legal practice. In his systematic and profoundly sensible way, Aristotle pointed out that it is a necessary condition that the cause be internal to the agent, but in addition, he characterized as involuntary the actions produced by coercion and actions produced in certain kinds of ignorance. As Aristotle well knew, however, no simple rule demarcates cases here. Clearly, some ignorance is not considered excusable, when it may be fairly judged that the agent should have known. Additionally, in some cases of coercion, the agent is expected to resist the pressure, given the nature of the situation. As Aristotle illustrates in his own discussion of such complexities, we seem to proceed to deal with these cases by judging their similarity to uncontroversial and well-worn prototypes. This run-of-the-mill cognitive strategy is reflected in the fundamental role that precedent law is accorded in determining subsequent judgments (see more extended explanations in PM Churchland 1995).

It is unlikely that there exists a sharp distinction between the voluntary and the involuntary – between being in control and being out of control – either in terms of behavioral conditions or in terms of the underlying neurobiology. The differences are differences in degree, not a clean bifurcation specified by necessary and sufficient conditions. An agent's decision to change television channels may be more in his control than his decision to pay for his child's college tuition, which may be more in his control than his decision to marry his wife, which may be more in his control than his decision to turn off the alarm clock. Some desires or fears may be very powerful, others less so, and we may have more self-control in some circumstances than in others. Hormonal changes, for example in puberty, make certain behavior patterns highly likely, and in general, the neurochemical milieu can have a powerful effect of the strength of desires, urges, drives and feelings.

As I shall suggest in below, however, at opposite ends of the self-control spectrum are prototypical cases that differ sufficiently in behavioral and internal features to provide a foundation for a basic, if somewhat rough-hewn, distinction between being in control and not, between being responsible and not. It will also be apparent as we reflect on the spectrum's end points that there are many parameters relevant to being in control. In our current state of neurobiological and behavioral knowledge, we do not know how to specify all those parameters. Nevertheless, we do know now that activity patterns in certain brain structures, including the amygdala, hypothalamus, somatosensory cortices, and ventromedial frontal cortex are important, and that levels of alleged neuromodulators, such as serotonin, dopamine, and norepinephrine, as well as hormones, play a critical role. Ultimately, as I shall explore later, a range of optimal values may be specifiable, and therewith, a contrasting range that is clearly sub-optimal.

Are We More In Control and More Responsible to the Degree That Emotions Play a Lesser Role and Reason Plays a Greater Role?

A view with deep historical roots assumes that, in matters of practical decision, reason and emotion are in opposition. To be in control, on this view, is to be maximally rational. To that end, one must maximize suppression of emotions, feelings, and inclinations. Emotion is considered the enemy of morality, and consequently moral judgment must be based on reason detached from emotion.

Immanuel Kant is the philosopher best known for adopting this view. In his moral philosophy, Kant saw human agents as attaining virtue only if as they succeed in downplaying feeling and inclination and giving reason complete control.[2] He says: "The rule and direction for knowing how you go about [making a decision],[3] without becoming unworthy of it, lies entirely in your reason." (from

---

[2] This is, needless to say, somewhat oversimplified.
[3] Kant actually says, "The rule and direction for knowing how you go about *sharing in happiness . . .*" (my italics) because the matter arises in the context of a teacher-student dialogue about a particular case, namely how to help others and whether to give them what they want. Pretty clearly Kant intends the point to be general, and hence my more general interpolation.

Fragments of a Moral Catechism 1797). In Kant's view, we would be perfectly rational save for the inclinations, feelings and desires based in our bodies. The perfect moral agent, Kant seems to suggest, is one whose decisions are perfectly rational and are detached entirely from emotion and feeling[4] (de Sousa calls such an agent a "Kantian monster;" de Sousa 1990, p. 14). The kinds of cases that inspire Kant's veneration of reason and his suspicion of the passions are the familiar "heart-over-head" blunders where the impassioned do-gooder makes things worse, when the long-term consequences were neglected while immediate need was responded to, when the fool does not look before he leaps. A powerful rationalist assumption underlies the great bulk of ethical theory in the latter half of this century. For example, the Kantian framework permeates the work of Nagel (1970), Rawls (1971), Gewirth (1978) and Donagan (1977).

Understanding the consequences of a plan, both its long- and short-term consequences, is obviously important, but is Kant right in assuming that feeling is the enemy of virtue, that moral education requires learning to disregard the bidding of inclination? Would we be more virtuous, or more educable morally, were we without passions, feelings, and inclinations?

Not according to David Hume, against whom Kant was probably reacting. Hume asserted that ". . . reason alone can never be a motive to any action of the will; and secondly, it can never oppose passion in the direction of the will" (p. 413). As he later explains: "T'is from the prospect of pain or pleasure that the aversion or propensity arises towards any object: And these emotions extend themselves to the causes and effects of that object, as they are pointed out to us by reason and experience" (p. 414). As Hume understands it, reason is responsible for delineating the various consequences of a plan, and thus reason and imagination work together to anticipate problems and payoffs. But feelings, informed by experience, are generated by the mind-brain in response to anticipations, and incline an agent towards or against a plan.

Common culture also finds something not quite right in the image of nonfeeling, nonemotional rationality. In the highly popular television series, Star Trek,[5] three of the main characters are portrayed as capable of varying degrees of emotional response. The pointy-eared semi-alien, Mr. Spock, is typified by the absence of emotion. In trying circumstances, his head is cool, his approach is calm. He faces catastrophe and narrow escape with easy-handed equanimity. He is puzzled by the humans' propensity to anger, fear, love and sorrow, and correspondingly fails to predict their appearance. Interestingly, Mr. Spock's cold reason sometimes results in bizarre decisions, even if they have a curious kind of "logic" to them.[6] By contrast, Dr. McCoy is found closer to the other end of the spectrum.

---

[4] Or as Marge Piercy remarks in Braided Lives (1982) ". . . treats his emotions like mice that infest our basement or rats in the garage, as vermin to be crushed in traps and poisoned with bait."

[5] This was originally broadcast in the 1960's. More recently, its successor, Start Trek – The Next Generation, has also been wildly popular. Spock has been replaced by the android, Data, who is largely without emotion, while Whorf, an alien who is "animalistic" and highly emotional, has also been included.

[6] Spock does not, however, resemble EVR in his decision-making (see below).

Individual human suffering inspires him to risk much, to ignore future costs, or to fly off the handle, often to Mr. Spock's taciturn evaluation, "but that's illogical." The balance between reason and emotion is more nearly epitomized by the legendary and beloved captain Kirk. By and large, his judgment is wise. He can make tough decisions when necessary, he can be merciful or courageous or angry, when appropriate. He is more nearly the ideal Aristotle identifies as the practically wise man.[7]

Neuropsychological studies are highly pertinent to the question of the significance of feeling in wise decision-making. Research by the Damasios and their colleagues on a number of patients with brain damage shows that, when deliberation is cut off from feelings, decisions are likely to be poor. Consider the patient SM whose amygdala has been destroyed and who lacks normal feelings of fear. She does not process fear signals normally, she does not recognize feelings of fear in herself, and does not evince normal facial expressions in fearful circumstances. SM does have a concept of fear of sorts, and she can tell when a human face shows a fear response. In complex circumstances, with no access to gut feelings of unease and fear, she is as likely as not to make a decision that normally wired people could easily foresee to be contrary to her interest. Whereas a normal subject would say he has an uneasy feeling about someone who is in fact predatorial, SM generates no such feelings. In a rather more complex way, the point is dramatically illustrated by the patient EVR, who first came to the Damasios' lab at the University of Iowa College of Medicine more than a decade ago.

A brain tumor in the ventromedial region of EVR's frontal lobes had been surgically removed earlier, leaving him with bilateral lesions. Following his surgery EVR enjoyed good recovery and seemed very normal, at least superficially. For example, he scored as well on standard IQ tests as he had before the surgery (about 140). He was knowledgeable, answered questions appropriately, and so far as mentation was concerned, seemed unscathed by his loss of brain tissue. EVR himself voiced no complaints. In his day-to-day life, however, a very different picture began to emerge. Once a steady, resourceful and efficient accountant, he now made a mess of his tasks, came in late, failed to finish easy jobs, and so forth. Once a reliable and loving family man, his personal life became a shambles. Because he scored well on IQ tests and because he was knowledgeable and bright, EVR's problems seemed to his physician more likely to be psychiatric than neurological. As we now know, this diagnosis turned out to be entirely wrong.

The case of EVR is by no means unique, and there are a number of patients with a similar lesion and a comparable behavioral profile. After studying EVR for some time, and comparing him to other cases of similar damage, the Damasios and their colleagues began to devise new tests to determine what about EVR's emotional responses were not in the normal range. For example, shown horrifying or disgusting pictures, his galvanic skin response (GSR)[8] was flat. Normals, in contrast, showed a huge response while viewing such pictures. On the other hand, he

---

[7] For an excellent discussion of faculty psychology, see Wittrup (1994).
[8] The GSR measures change in conductivity of the skin as a function of increased sweat on the skin, which is an effect produced by the sympathetic system of the nervous system.

could feel fear or pleasure in uncomplicated, more basic, situations. During the following years, new and more revealing tests were devised to try and probe more precisely the relation between reasoning logically on the one hand, and acting in accordance with reason on the other. For there was no doubt that EVR could evince the correct answer to questions concerning what would be the best action to take (e.g., defer a small gratification now for a larger reward later), but his own behavior often conflicted with his stated convictions (e.g., he would seize the small reward now, missing out on the large reward later; Saver and Damasio 1991).

Antoine Bechara, working with the Damasios, developed a particularly revealing test. In this test, a subject is presented with four decks of cards and told that his task is to make as much profit as possible, given an initial loan of money. Subjects are told to turn over cards, one at a time, from any of the four decks. They are not told how many cards can be played (a series of 100) or what the payoffs are from any deck. One has to discover everything by trial and error. After turning over each card, the subjects are rewarded with an amount of money, and on some cards, they may also be penalized and be required to pay out money. Behind the scenes, the experimenter designates two decks, C and D, to be low-paying ($50) and to contain some moderate penalty cards; two other decks, A and B, pay large amounts ($100) but contain very high penalty cards. Things are rigged so that players incur a net loss if they play mostly A and B, but do well if they play mostly C and D decks. Subjets cannot calculate exactly their losses and gains, because there is too much mentally to keep track of. Instead, subjects must generate a sense of what strategy will work to their advantage.

During the game, normal controls come fairly quickly to stick mainly with low-paying, low-penalty decks (C and D) and make a profit. What is striking is that subjects such as EVR (ventromedial frontal damage) tend to end with a loss because they choose mainly high-paying decks despite the profit-eating penalty cards. Subjects with brain damage to regions other than ventromedial behave like controls. As Bechara et al. (1994) note, even after repeated testing on the task as long as a month later or as soon as twenty-four hours later, EVR continued to play heavily the losing decks. When queried at the end of the trial, he verbally reported that A and B were losing decks. To put it rather paradoxically, rationally EVR does indeed know what the best long-run strategy is, but in exercising choice in actual action, he goes for short-run gain, incurring long-run loss. Is EVR merely showing frontal perseveration? No, because he does score normally on the Wisconsin card-sorting task, in contrast to perseverative patients. In any case, he does sometimes try other decks. To make matters more difficult for the Kantian ideal, his judgments of recency and frequency are flawless, his knowledge base and short-term memory are intact (Bechara et al. 1994). Moreover, EVR can articulate well enough the future consequences of alternative actions, so the problem cannot be lack of understanding of what might happen. In sum, what seems chiefly to be amiss here is not EVR's capacity to reason; rather, it is the inability of emotions to affect his reason and decision-making.

That his "pure reasoning," displayed verbally, and his "practical decision-making," displayed in choice, were so at odds suggested to the Damasios that the real problem lay with EVR's lack of emotional responsivity to situations that involved some understanding of the meaning and implications of the events. This is consistent with his lack of skin response while viewing emotionally charged photographs. That is, although EVR would react normally to simple conditions such as a loud noise or a threat of attack, he failed to respond in more complex situations whose significance might involve more subtle or culturally mediated features, such as the social consequences of failure to complete jobs or the future consequences of a sudden marriage to a prostitute or profit-making in the Bechara gambling task. EVR and similar subjects seem to have a kind of insensitivity to the significance of future consequences, whether they are rewarding, as in the gambling task, or punishing, as in a reverse gambling task. This insensitivity seems best understood in terms of the failure to provide a "value mark," via somatic states, to the various options (Bechara et al. 1994; Damasio 1994; Adolphs et al., this volume).

Further results came from the analysis of skin conductance data taken by a galvanometer placed on the arm of each subject during the gambling task (Damasio et al. 1995). In the gambling task, neither controls nor frontal patients showed a skin response to card selections in the first few plays of the game (selections 1–10). By about the tenth selection, however, controls began to exhibit a skin response immediately prior to begining to reach for the "bad" decks. When queried at this stage about how they were making their choices, controls (and frontal patients) said they had no idea whatever, they were just exploring. By about selection 20, controls continued to get a consistent skin response just before reaching for the "bad" decks. In their verbal reports, controls said that they still did not know what was the best strategy, but that they had a feeling that maybe decks A and B were "funny." By selection 50, controls typically could articulate, and follow, the winning strategy. Frontal patients never did show a skin response in reaching for any deck. What is so striking here is that in controls, good choice was in some measure biased by the feeling even before subjects were aware of the feeling, and well before they could articulate the winning strategy. That many of our daily choices are likewise biased without our being aware of the feeling seems altogether likely.[9]

The significance for choice of feeling, and of unaware biasing by feeling, has implications for the economists' favored model of "rational choice." According to this model, the ideally rational (wise) agent begins deliberation by laying out all alternatives, calculating the expected utility for each alternative based on probability of each outcome multiplied by the value of (goodies accruing to) each outcome. He ends by choosing the alternative with the highest expected utility score. In light of the data just considered, this model seems highly unsatisfactory. At best, it probably applies to a small range of highly quanitifable problems, but even then comes into play after "cognition-cum-feeling" brings to awareness the restricted set of "feels-reasonable" alternatives. At any rate, the economists' model is unlikely to come even close to giving the whole story of rational choice.

---

[9] Benjamin Libet came to a similar conclusion using a very different experimental paradigm (Libet 1985).

A major idea in the Damasios' work on decision-making is that representation of changes in body state, comprising visceral feeling as well as musculoskeletal signals (both external 'touch' sensations and sympathetic system changes in skin), play an essential role in biasing choice.[10] Body-state representation systematically integrates diverse changes in information originating in the sympathetic system. As future plans and possible-plans develop, the imagination generates representations of plan sequelae, and to these, as well as to perceptually driven representations, visceral responses are generated, via mediation of the amygdala and hypothalamus. Somewhat more elaborately, therefore, the Damasios envisage a complex to-ing and fro-ing of signals between thalamo-cortical states and changes in the body as being the crucial pathways for self-representation and for sensible decision-making.

The connection between this hypothesis and the case of EVR and others with similar lesions (ventromedial frontal) is obvious. The point is not that EVR-type patients feel nothing at all. Rather, it is that in those situations requiring imaginative elaboration of the consequences of an option, feelings are not generated in response to the imagined scenario. This is because the ventromedial frontal region needed for integration of body-state representation and fancy "scenario-spinning" is disconnected from the "gut feelings." Normally, neurons in ventromedial frontal cortex would project to and from areas such as the amygdala and hypothalamus that contain neurons carrying body-state signals. In patients with destruction of ventromedial cortex, the pathways are disrupted.

It is this set of complex responses, involving future-consequences recognition, visceral changes, and feelings, that the Damasios see as inclining the person to one decision rather than another. That is, in the context of acquired cognitive-cum-emotional understanding about the world, neuronal activity in these pathways biases sensible decisions. Moreover, the biasing can begin before subjects are aware of it, and before they can articulate their inclinations, even though a particular decision may seem, introspectively, to be the outcome solely of conscious deliberation. Their hypothesis is that when EVR is confronted with a question ("should I finish this job or watch the football game?"; "should I choose from deck A or from deck C?"), his brain's body-state representation contains nothing about changes in the viscera, and hence he is missing important biasing clues that something is foolish or unwise or problematic. His frontal lobes, needed for a complex decision, have no access to information about the valence of a complex situation or plan or idea. Therefore, some of EVR's behavior turns out to be foolish and unreasonable (for a comprehensive account, see AR Damasio's 1994 book, Descartes' Error: Emotion, Reason and The Human Brain).

---

[10] An earlier hypothesis related to this view was suggested by Paul MacLean (1949,1952). He said "As a working hypothesis, it can be inferred that the limbic system is for the "body viscous", a visceral brain that interprets and gives expression to its incoming information in terms of feeling . . ." (1952). See also James Papez (1937), H Kluver and PC Bucy (1937, 1938).

Are There Significant Neurobiological Differences Between "In Control" Agents and "Out of Control" Agents?

I am assuming there is a real difference in what we may loosely call "life success" between agents whose behavior is generally at the "in control" end of the spectrum – agents typified by the fictional Captain Kirk – and on the other hand, agents whose behavior is often at the "out of control" end of the spectrum, typified by the obsessive-compulsive subject. To a first approximation, the behavior of the "in controls" is more conducive to their interests, long- and short-term, and they generally make sensible, reasonable, and wise decisions about both short- and long-term plans. Undoubtedly the relevant behavioral differences cannot be simply reduced to a formula for "reproductive fitness" or even "inclusive fitness," yet they are almost certainly deeply related to properties sensitive to natural selection. Are there likely to be prototypical neurobiological differences that correlate with these behavioral differences, vaguely specified though they are? Is it possible to provide an outline of the neurobiology prototypes at either end of our "in control/ out of control" spectrum, based on the empirical data so far?

In a rather crude, semi-speculative, and somewhat metaphorical way, yes. Having made all those hedges, let me now be a bit bolder. To begin with, converging data from neuropsychological research, animal studies and anatomy implicate certain brain structures as especially crucial in emotional response. Assuming the Damasio hypothesis is largely correct, these structures are presumably essential for "in control" behavior. So far, the list of structures include the amygdala, somatosensory cortical areas I and II, insula, hypothalamus, anterior cingulate cortex, basal ganglia and ventromedial frontal region of cortex. That there is more than one area indicates that "control," in this vague sense, is probably a distributed function in which a number of structures participate. The aforementioned structures also heavily project to and from each other. We also know that the connectivity between these regions is essential to normal functioning, as evidenced by subjects such as EVR, SM and others. Given the data, therefore, it may be expected that certain general dynamical properties of the neural networks in these regions probably characterize functioning in the normal range. How might we begin to specify the dynamical properties typical of the normal range?

The brain is a complex dynamical system. If we consider the brain's neurons as defining axes in a multidimensional state space, neuronal activity can be represented as points in the state space, and patterns of neuronal activity as trajectories in that state space. Additionally, trajectories can be linked to make sequences of trajectories in that state space. Planning for a future contingency, for example how to portage around heavy rapids or how to convince a jury of Simpson's guilt, involves putting together a long and complex sequence of trajectories, first in imagination and later in behavior. Given available data, it seems reasonable to assume that the "well-tempered" brain of a person who is typically wise, sensible and reasonable embodies a kind of stable landscape in that state space. This means, among other things, that trajectories, appropriate to the sensory environment, through that state space, are highly stable to small perturbations. On the other hand, when the structures are damaged by lesions or by highly abnormal changes in neurochemical milieu, the landscape of the state space changes, and the trajectories become unstable and bizarre. To use a related analogy, the limit cycle characterizing the stable path in neuronal space can suddenly be replaced by very different, and behaviorally inappropriate, limit cycles.

Certain general features of the "neuronal landscape" may be particularly dependent on the neurochemicals of the widely projecting systems, such as those involving serotonin, dopamine, or norepinephrine (Fig. 1). When the concentrations of these chemicals change by a certain threshold, they may quite radically change the terrain of the landscape, for example by flattening it to make trajectories more susceptible to perturbations, or digging deep grooves that are hard to get out of even when the environment calls for a different trajectory. The widely projecting systems appear to play a role in modulating the responses of neurons, for example, by changing the gain or by down-regulating responsivity to neurotransmitters such as glutamate. They appear to play a crucial role in sleep and dreaming, in attention, and in mood, and they are found in brain stem structures that diffusely project to cortical and subcortical structures. We do not, however, understand in detail the interactions between these systems, nor exactly how changing their concentrations changes the neuronal landscape.

What is known at the behavioral level is that obsessive-compulsive disorder (OCD), for example, is very treatable by serotonin agonists such as fluoxetine (Prozac); patients gain control over their phobias and their compulsive behavior. It is well known that many cases of medical depression respond extremely well to drugs that enhance serotonin or norepinephrine, giving patients control over their anger and lassitude. Tourette's syndrome is much more controlled when patients are given serotonin agonists. Each of these interventions can be seen, in keeping with the favored metaphor, as establishing or re-establishing general features in neuronal landscape that make it stable against noise and perturbation, while allowing exploration and innovation without wild deviation from the stable trajectories.

Research from basic neuroscience as well as from lesion studies and scan studies will be needed to transform this speculative outline into a substantial, detailed, testable account of the general features of the landscape that are typical of "in control" subjects. These dynamical systems properties may be quite abstract, for "in control" individuals may differ in temperament and in cognitive strategies (see Kagan 1994). As Aristotle might have put it, there are different ways to harmonize the soul. Nevertheless, the prediction is that, at the very least, some such general features probably are specifiable. It is relatively easy to see that dynamical systems properties do distinguish between brains that perform certain tasks, such as walking well or poorly. What I am proposing here is that more abstract skills that are characterizable behaviorally, such as being a successful shepherd dog or a competent lead sled dog, can also be specified in terms of dynamical systems properties, dependent as they are on neural networks and neurochemical concentrations. My hunch is that human skills in planning, prepar-

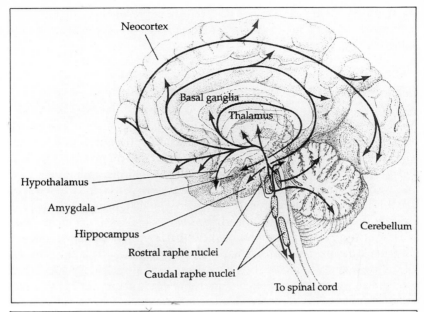

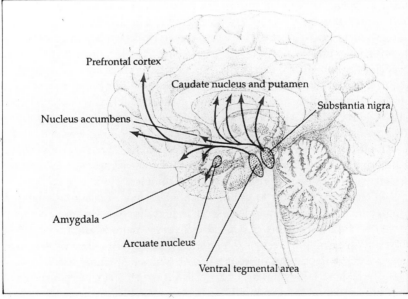

Fig. 1. A A schematic illustration of the projection patterns of neurons containing serotonin (5-HT) whose cell bodies are located in the chain of raphe nuclei lying along the midline of the brainstem. Within each region receiving a projection, there are many axon terminals (reprinted with permission from Nicholls et al. 1992). **B** A schematic illustration of the projection pattern of neurons containing dopamine whose cell bodies are located in nuclei of the hypothalamus (reprinted with permission from Nicholls et al. 1992)

ing and co-operating can likewise be specified, not now, not next year, but in the fullness of time as neuroscience and experimental psychology develop and flourish.

Learning What Is Rational and What Is Not

Aristotle would have us add here the point that there is an important relation between self-control and habit formation. A substantial part of learning to cope with the world, to defer gratification, to show anger and compassion appropriately, and to have courage when necessary involves acquiring appropriate decision-making habits. In the metaphor of dynamical systems, this is interpreted as sculpting the terrain of the neuronal state space so that behaviorally appropriate trajectories are well-grooved. Clearly, we have much to learn about what this consists of, both at the behavioral and neuronal levels. We do know, however, that if an infant has damage in some of the critical regions, such as the ventromedial frontal cortex or amygdala, then typical acquisition of the right "Aristotelian" contours may be next to impossible, and more direct intervention may sometimes be necessary to achieve what normal children routinely achieve as they grow up.

The characterization of a choice or an action as "rational" carries a strongly normative component, implying, for example, that it was in one's long range interest, or in the long range interest of some relevantly specified group, or not inconsistent with other things one believes or what is believed by "reasonable" people. It is not sheerly descriptive, in contrast, for example, to describing the action as performed clumsily or with a hammer. Claiming an action was rational often carries the implication that the choice was conducive in some significant way to the agent's interests or well-being or to those of his family, and that it properly took into account the consequences of the action, both long- and short-term (see also Johnson 1993); thus the evaluative component. Though a brief dictionary definition can capture some salient aspects of what it means to be rational and reasonable, it hardly does justice to the real complexity of the concept.

As children, we learn to evaluate actions as more or less rational by being exposed to prototypical examples, as well as to prototypical examples of foolish or unwise or irrational actions. Insofar as we learn by example, learning about rationality is like learning to recognize patterns in general, whether it be recognizing what is a dog, what is food, or when a person is afraid or embarrassed or weary. As Paul Churchland (1995) has argued, we also learn ethical concepts such as "fair" and "unfair," "kind" and "unkind," by being shown prototypical cases and generalizing to novel but relevantly similar situations.[11] Now as we know, learning from examples is something networks do exceedingly well. Peer and parental feedback hone the pattern recognition network so that, over time, it comes to closely resem-

---

[11] In his splendid book, Moral Imagination (1993), Mark Johnson argues for a similar view. See also Owen Flanagan's excellent book (1991), Varieties of Moral Personality: Ethics and Psychological Realism.

ble the standard in the wider community. Nevertheless, as Socrates was fond of showing, articulating those standards is a hopeless task, even when a person successfully uses the expression "rational," case by case. Making an algorithm for rational choice is almost certainly impossible. The systematic failure of artificial intelligence research to discover how to program computers to conform to common sense is an indication of the profoundly nonalgorithmic nature of common sense, rationality and practical wisdom.

This is important because most philosophers regard the evaluative dimension of ethical concepts to imply that their epistemology must be entirely different from that of descriptive concepts. What appears to be special about learning some concepts, such as "rational," "impractical" and "fair," is only that the basic wiring for feeling the appropriate emotion must be intact. That is, the prototypical situation of something being impractical or shortsighted typically arouses unpleasant feelings of dismay and concern; the prospect of something being dangerous arouses feelings of fear, and these feelings, along with perceptual features, are probably an integral part of what is learned in perceptual pattern recognition.

Simple dangerous situations – crossing a busy street, encountering a grizzly with cubs – can probably be learned as dangerous without the relevant feelings. At least that is suggested by the evidence of the Damasios from their patient SM who, you may recall, suffered amygdala destruction and lacks normal fear processing. Although she can identify which simple situations are dangerous, this seems for her to be a purely cognitive, nonaffective judgment. However, her recognition is poor when she needs to detect the menace or hostility or pathology in complex social situations, where no simple formula for identifying danger is available. As suggested earlier, the appropriate feelings may be necessary for skilled application of a concept, if not for fairly routine applications. This is perhaps why the fictional Mr. Spock, lacking emotions as he is, is poor at predicting what will provoke strong sympathy or dread or embarrassment in humans.

Stories, both time-honored as well as those passing as local gossip, provide a basic core of scenarios where children imagine and feel, if vicariously, the results of various choices, such as failing to prepare for future hard times (The Ant and The Grasshopper) or failing to heed warnings (The Boy Who Cried Wolf), of being conned by a smooth talker (Jack and the Beanstock), of vanity in appearance (Narcissus). As children, we can vividly feel and imagine the foolishness of trying to please everybody (The Old Man and his Donkey), of not caring to please anybody (Scrooge in Dickens' A Christmas Carol), and of pleasing the "wrong" people (the prodigal son). Many of the great and lasting stories, for example by Shakespeare, Ibsen, Tolstoy, Balzac, are rife with moral ambiguity, reflecting the fact that real life is rife with conflicting feeling and emotions, and that simple foolishness is far easier to avoid than great tragedy. Buridan's dithering ass was just silly; Hamlet's ambivalence and hesitation was deeply tragic and all too understandable. In the great stories is also a reminder that our choices are always made amidst a deep and unavoidable ignorance of many of the details of the future, where coping with that very uncertainty is something about which one can be more or less wise. For all decisions save the trivial ones, there is no algorithm for making a wise choice (see again Johnson 1993; Flanagan 1991). As for matters such as choosing a career or a mate, having children or not, moving to a certain place or not, deciding the guilt or innocence of a person on trial, etc., these are usually complex constraint satisfaction problems.

As we deliberate about a choice, we are guided by – and guide others by – our reflection on past deeds, our recollection of pertinent stories, and our imagining of the sequence of effects that would be brought about by choosing one option or another. Antonio Damasio calls the feelings generated in the imagining-deliberating context "secondary emotions" (Damasio 1994, p. 134 ff.) to indicate that they are a response not to external stimuli, but to internally generated representations and recollections. As we learn and grow up, we come to associate certain feelings with certain types of situation, and this combination can be reactivated when a similar set of conditions arises. Often a moral dilemma cannot be easily labeled, and instead we draw analogies between types of dilemmas: "this is like the time my father got lost in the blizzard and built a quinze;" "this is like the time Clarence Darrow defended a teacher's right to teach evolutionary biology," etc. Recognition of a present situation as relevantly like a certain past case has, of course, a cognitive dimension, but it also evokes feelings that are similar to those evoked by the past case, and this is important in aiding the cortical network to relax into a solution concerning what to do next.

What Happens to the Concept of Responsibility?

We need now to return to the dominant background question motivating this essay. One very general conclusion is provoked by the foregoing discussion. On the whole, social groups work best when individuals are considered responsible agents, and hence as a matter of practical life, it is probably wisest to hold mature agents responsible for their behavior and for their habits. That is, it is probably in everyone's interest if the default assumption in place is that agents have control over their actions and that, in general, agents are liable to punishment and praise for their actions. This is of course a highly complex and subtle issue, but the basic idea is that feeling the social consequences of one's choices is a critical part of socialization, of learning to be in the give and take of the group. (This pragmatic point of view, most closely associated with the ideas of Spinoza (1677), can also be found in the classic essays of Hobart (1934) and Schlick (1939).) Feeling those consequences is necessary for contouring the state space landscape in the appropriate way, and that means feeling the approval and disapproval meted out. A child must learn about the physical world by interacting with it and bearing the consequences of its actions, or watching others engage the world, or hearing about how others engage the world. As with social animals generally, learning about the social world involves cognitive-affective learning, directly or indirectly, about the nature of the social consequences of a choice. This must, of course, be consistent with reasonably protecting the developing child, and with compassion, kindness and understanding. In short, I do not want the simplicity of the general conclusion to mask the tremendous subtleties of child-rearing. Underlying all the necessary subtlety, however, the basic pragmatist point is just this: if the only known way for "social decency" circuitry to develop requires that the subject generate the relevant feelings pursuant to social pattern recognition, and if that, in turn, requires experiences of praise (pleasure) and blame (pain) consequent upon his actions, then treating the agent as responsible for behavior is a pragmatically justified operating assumption. That is, it is justified by its practical necessity.

This of course leaves it open that, under special circumstances, agents should be excused from responsibility or accorded diminished responsibility. In general, the law courts are struggling, case by case, to make reasonable judgments about what those circumstances are, and no simple rule really works. Neuropsychological data are clearly relevant here, as for example in cases where the subjects' brains show an anatomical resemblance to the brain of EVR or SM. Quite as obviously, however, the data do not show that no one is ever really responsible and deserving of punishment or praise. Nor do they show that, when life is hard, one is entitled to avoid responsibility.

Is direct intervention in the circuitry morally acceptable? This too is a hugely complex and infinitely ramifying issue. My personal bias is twofold: first, that in general, at any level, be it ecosystem or immune system, intervening in biology always requires great caution. When the target of the intervention is the nervous system, then caution by many more orders of magnitude is wanted. Still, not taking action is nevertheless doing something, and acts of omission can be every bit as consequential as acts of commission. Second, the movie, Clockwork Orange, immediately associated with the very idea of direct intervention in criminal law, probably had a greater impact on our collective amygdaloid structures than it deserves to have. Certainly some kinds of direct intervention are morally objectionable. So much is easy. But all kinds? Even pharmacological? Is it possible that some forms of nervous system intervention might be more humane than lifelong incarceration or death? It seems to me likely that the general answer is yes. I do not know the detailed answers to these questions but, given what we now understand about the role of emotion in reason, perhaps the time has come to give them a careful, calm and thorough reconsideration. Guided by Aristotle, we may say that these are, au fond, pragmatic questions concerning the well-functioning of certain social animals, namely hominids.

Conclusions

I have considered three vintage philosophical theses in the context of new data from neuroscience: 1) feelings are an essential component of viable practical reasoning about what to do (David Hume); 2) moral agents come to be morally and practically wise not by dint of "pure cognition", but by developing through life experiences the appropriate cognitive-connative habits (Aristotle); and 3) agents need to acquire the cognitive-connative skills to evaluate the consequences of certain events and the price of taking risks, and hence must be treated as responsible agents (Hobart 1934; Schlick 1939). Each of the theses has been controversial and remains so now; each has been the target of considerable philosophical criticism. Now, however, as the data come in from neuropsychology as well as experimental psychology and basic neuroscience, the empirical probability of each seems evident. One may interpret Damasio's book, Descartes' Error, as the beginning of a neurobiological perspective on the ideas of Aristotle and Hume. In this evolving scientific context, many important social policy questions must be considered afresh, including those concerned with the most efficacious means, consistent with other human values, for achieving civil harmony. Much, much more, of course, needs to be learned, for example about the reward circuits in the brain, about pleasure and anxiety and fear. Philosophically, the emphasis with respect to civic, personal, and intellectual virtue has been focused almost exclusively on the purely cognitive domain, with affective domain largely left out of the equation, as though the Kantian conception of reasoning and choice were in fact correct. In matters of education and social policy, how best to factor in feeling and affect is something requiring a great deal of mulling, and practical wisdom. In any case, my hope is that understanding more about the empirical facts of decision-making, both at the neuronal level and the behavioral level, may be useful as we aim for practical wisdom and ponder issues of social policy.

Acknowledgments. I am particularly indebted to Hanna Damasio and Antonio Damasio for extended discussions on these and related topics. I wish also to thank Francis Crick, Paul Churchland, Rodolfo Llinas, David Brink, Deborah Forster, Jordan Hughes, Philip Kitcher, Laura Reider, and the members of the Experimental Philosophy Lab at UCSD.

References

Aristotle. The Nichomachean Ethics. translated by JAK Thompson (1955) Harmondsworth: Penguin Books

Bechara A, Damasio AR, Damasio H, Anderson SW (1994) Insensitivity to future consequences following damage to human prefrontal cortex. Cognition 50:7–15

Campbell CA (1957) On selfhood and godhood. London; George Allen and Unwin Ltd, and New Jersey; Humanities Press Inc., pp 158–179

Cheney DL, Seyfarth RM (1990) How Monkeys See the World. Chicago, University of Chicago Press

Churchland Paul M (1995) The engine of reason. The seat of the soul. Cambridge, MA, MIT Press

Clutton-Brock TH, Parker GA (1995) Punishment in animal societies. Nature 373:209–216

Crick F (1994) The Astonishing Hypothesis. New York, Scribners

Damasio A (1994) Descartes' Error: Emotion, Reason and The Human Brain. New York, Grosset/Putnam

Damasio AR, Tranel D, Damasio H (1991) Somatic markers and the guidance of behavior. In: Levin H, Eisenberg H, Benton A (eds) Frontal lobe function and dysfunction. New York, Oxford University Press

De Sousa R (1990) The rationaligy of emotion. Cambridge, MA, MIT Press

de Waal FBM (1982) Chimpanzee politics. London, Allen and Unwin

Donagan A (1977) The theory of morality. Chicago; Chicago University Press

de Waal FBM (1989) Dominance 'style' and primate social organization. In: Standen V, Foley R (eds) Comparative socioecology: the behavioral ecology of humans and other mammals. Oxford, Blackwells

Flanagan O (1991) Varieties of moral personality: ethics and Psychological realism. Cambridge, Harvard Univcersity Press

Gewrith A (1978) Reason and morality. Chicago, Chicago University Press

Hobart RE (1934) Free will as involving determinism and inconceivable without it. Mind 43:1–27

Hume D (1739) A treatise of human nature. Edited by LA Selby-Bigge as Hume's Treatise. Oxford, Oxford University Press

Johnson M (1993) Moral imagination. Chicage, Chicago University Press

Kagan J (1994) Galen's prophecy: temperament in human nature. New York, Basic Books

Kant I (1797) Fragments of a moral catechism. In: The metaphysical principles of virtue, translated by James Ellington (1964). New York, Bobbs-Merrill, 148–53

Kenny AJP (1989). The metaphysics of mind. Oxford, Clarendon Press

Kluver H and Bucy PC (1937) "Psychic blindness", and other symptoms following bilateral temporal lobectomy in rhesus monkeys. Am J Physiol 119:352–352

Kluver H, Bucy PC (1938) An analysis of certain effects of bilateral temporal lobectomy in the rhesus monkey, with special reference to "psychic blindness". J Psychol 5:33–54

Libet B (1985) Unconscious cerebral initiative and the role of conscious will in voluntary action. Behav Brain Sci 8:529–566

MaClean PD (1949) Psychosomatic disease and the "visceral brain." Recent developments on the Papez theory of emotion. Psychosomatic Med 11:338–353

MacLean PD (1952) Some psychiatric implications of physiological studies on frontotemporal portion of limbic system (visceral brain). Electrophysiol Clin Neurophysiol 4:407–418

Nagel T (1970) The possibility of altruism. Princeton, NJ, Princeton University Press

Nicholls JG, Martin AR, Wallace BG (1992) From neuron to brain. Sunderland MA, Sinauer Associates

Papez JW (1937) A proposed mechanism of emotion. Arch Neurol Psychiat 38:725–744

Piercy M (1982) Braided lives. New York, Knopf

Rawls J (1971) A theory of justice. Cambridge, MA, Harvard University Press

Saver JL, Damasio AR (1991) Preserved access and processing of social knowledge in a patient with acquired sociopathy due to ventromedial frontal damage. Neuropsychologia 29:1241–1249

Schlick M (1939) When is a man responsible? In: Problems of ethics, translated by David Rynin. New York, Prentice-Hall, 143–156

Taylor R (1974) Metaphysics. Englewood Cliffs, NJ, Prentice-Hall Inc

Spinoza B (1677) Ethics. Republished in The Collected Works of Spinoza (1985 E Curley ed). Princeton, NJ: Princeton University Press

Wittrup E (1994) A mind with a heart of its own. Ph.D. dissertation for UCSD, unpublished

Epilogue: Models of Decision-Making

J. Altman

In 1987, my colleague Jenny Kien and I published a paper entitled, "A model for decision making in the insect nervous system" (Altman and Kien 1987a). At that time, neurobiologists were paying virtually no attention to the process of choosing or selecting actions, although we subsequently discovered the papers by Damasio et al. describing EVR, a patient with damage to the ventro-medial frontal lobes who was unable to make decisions (see Damasio 1994). From these small seeds the flourishing bush described by the papers in this volume has sprung.

Our thesis in 1987 was that decision-making is a central and continuous part of the neural control of behaviour, from single neurons through simple circuits to whole systems; this is a view now gaining acceptance, as reflected by many of the present authors (see also Kien et al. 1992). In this final chapter, I will briefly explore how this model and its subsequent developments (Altman and Kien 1989; Nutzel et al. 1994; Kien and Altman 1995) apply to some of the aspects of decision-making in primates discussed elsewhere in this volume.

The original model (Fig. 1a) was a descriptive network based on research into control of walking and flight in insects. The output at any moment is selected by the activity in the whole network and results from a consensus between the activity in several intensively interconnected stations (N_1, N_2, and N_3) and their inputs. The inputs derive from novel changes in the environment (A), the internal state of the animal (C), which includes its past history, and re-afference, both between stations (X, Y, Z) and through the animal's action on its environment (B). (Mechanical limitations imposed by the design of the body (D) are discussed below.) The model is not homogeneous because the stations are connected in parallel loops, each with its own function (Altman and Kien 1987a,b, 1989; Kien and Altman 1992a,b). The consensus that determines the output is thus essentially the across-fibre pattern of activity in all the loops at any moment.

The emerging picture of the functional organisation of the prefrontal lobes, discussed by several authors in this volume, bears considerable similarity to this model. Pandya and Yeterian emphasise that the functions classically ascribed to the prefrontal lobes depend on its heavy interconnections with other parts of the cortex and with subcortical structures, such as the basal ganglia and limbic system. Fuster goes on to stress that the brain has no centre for will or for making choices; instead, decisions result from the interactions between these many brain areas

37D, Lordship Park, London N16 5UN, UK

A.R. Damasio et al. (Eds.)
Neurobiology of Decision-Making
© Springer-Verlag Berlin Heidelberg 1996

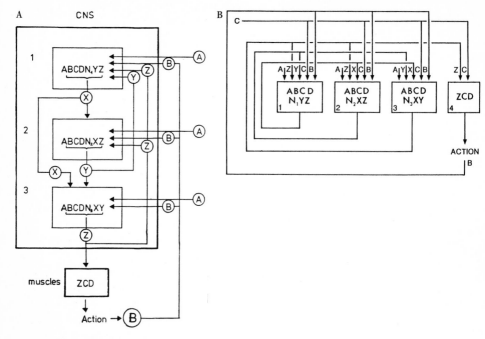

Fig. 1. Two versions of a model for deciding what to do at any instant. In both models, changes in any of the inputs result in changes in the output, whose nature depends on the state of the whole network at that moment. **A** A descriptive model for decision-making, based on research into the neural control of walking and flying in insects (modified from Altman and Kien 1987). The three stations (1–3) represent three ganglionic structures in the insect nervous system (1 = brain, 2 = suboesophageal ganglion, 3 = segmental ganglia) but the model can also be applied to equivalent centres in the mammalian nervous system, e.g., cortex, brain stem and spinal cord. For further explanation, see text. **B** The model in **A** redrawn as an attractor neural network (modified from Altman and Kien 1989; reproduced with permission from Kien and Altman 1995)

whose inputs converge in the prefrontal lobes. Neither are the prefrontal lobes homogeneous: their connections form a number of loops, reflecting subdivisions of function, with the dorso-lateral area involved in working (or active) memory, attention and planning, while the ventro-medial area deals with decision-making in social contexts (Pandya, Fuster, H. Damasio, A. Damasio).

Another significant feature of our model is that it stresses the importance of context in decision-making. Context is not just the external situation the animal finds itself in, but includes its own internal state at the time. This is why the findings reported by A. Damasio, Adolphs and their colleagues are so exciting, for they demonstrate how essential for competent decision-making are internal signals, which Damasio calls somatic markers (experienced as emotions or "gut feelings").

Somatic markers provide one of several mechanisms that limit the choices open to the animal at a given moment, sparing the need to carry maps of all eventualities or to unfold innumerable scenarios for all possible options. Another limit, described by Berthoz, is the matching of available information to an internal repertoire of patterns for evaluating motor choices. On top of these short-term constraints are, as several authors remark, limits set by the design of the body (D in Fig. 1), by the nerve circuits selected by evolution and by the animal's own history (see also Altman and Kien 1987a; Kien and Altman 1995).

More recent developments of our model have provided both informal and formal descriptions of this restriction of choices, which becomes particularly important when considering the sequences of actions that make up a behaviour (see below). Because the outputs from each station feed back into the network, the model belongs to the general class known as attractor neural networks (ANN; Fig. 1b; Altman and Kien 1989). ANNs continuously adjust their outputs according to the input and feedback signals they receive, until they reach a stable pattern of activity across the whole network, known as an attractor. We consider an ANN relaxing into an attractor the equivalent of the nervous system making a decision; the conditions in the network at the time determine what the choice will be.

Making a choice restricts the range of options available; deciding to walk to work instead of driving limits the choice of actions to be performed. One picture that gives an analogy of this process is the selection of a particular view through a zoom lens (Kien and Altman 1995); once the scene is selected, its components can be examined in greater detail. Another description is the "probability landscape" (Kien and Altman 1995), where the current input conditions form hills and valleys. The valleys represent a high probability that a particular output will occur. Entering a large valley is equivalent to selecting a particular behaviour; this restricts the choice to the smaller hollows within it, which represent the selection of actions needed to carry the behaviour out. As the inputs change, partly as the results of ongoing activity, the conformation of the landscape changes; the original valley may flatten out and new valleys appear that provide other choices.

The network relaxing into an attractor is the equivalent of entering a valley in the probability landscape. The ANN model shows that attractors are reached as a result of the total pattern of activity in the network. Although a single strong input may dominate the pattern, a combination of weaker inputs could be more powerful. A small change in an input can have a large effect if it comes at the right moment (Kien and Altman 1995).

For this reason, I am worried by the terms "winner-take-all/winner-lose-all" used by Fuster and Sejnowski to characterise the competition between inputs that determines the outputs from, respectively, the prefrontal lobes and basal ganglia. "Winner" to me implies the strongest input and thus conjures up shades of the old command fibre hypothesis (Kupfermann and Weiss 1978). Finding the right word is particularly important to capture the operational principles where population coding and neuronal ensembles are involved, as is likely here. We use the word "consensus" (Kien 1983), which is also imprecise for it implies general agreement, to describe the output that emerges from the overall pattern of the inputs. In this across-fibre pattern, at any moment some inputs are silent, some excitatory, some inhibitory, and the pattern changes continually as the behaviour progresses

(Altman and Kien 1987a). Where there is competition between inputs, it might be better to think in terms of a "winning combination" in the pattern of activity determining the output.

This difficulty points up a dislocation between how we think about and describe the process of decision-making and the actual operations that may be at work in the nervous system. Subjectively, it seems that choices are made, courses of action selected. In our descriptive model we have a CHOOSE-and-COMPARE process. Yet in the attractor networks there is no choice or selection; the output is a result of the overall pattern of activity, the relaxation towards an attractor. CHOOSE-and-COMPARE is simply the state of the network at any moment. If the operations of the nervous system are in any way similar to those of an ANN, we do not need to search for mechanisms of choice; there may be no winners in the nervous system, only outputs.

Ultimately, decision-making is not about single choices but about plans for achieving goals, which brings in the dimension of time. Recently we extended our model to describe the temporal relationship between the functional levels involved in executing such plans (Kien and Altman 1995). Fuster describes the prefrontal lobes setting up the overall plan of an action, the premotor cortex dealing with sequence of movements and the primary motor cortex organising single movements. Although these levels – which we call behaviour, routine and movement, respectively – form a functional hierarchy, our model shows that the actions they contain happen simultaneously, not sequentially. Walking (routine) is a series of steps (movements), each a sequence of muscle contractions. Each level can be considered as a time frame, nested in the levels above and with the levels below nested in it, best illustrated as several concentric circles (Fig. 2). The radius sweeping round the circle represents what is happening at any moment.

Once a behaviour has been selected, it has to be maintained until its goal or aim is fulfilled. Selection and maintenance are in fact a unitary process that we call CHOOSE-and-COMPARE, which runs until the current input conditions match an

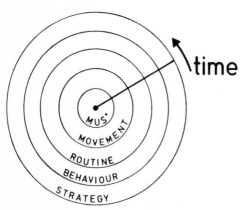

Fig. 2. Functional levels of activity in the nervous system form time frames, shown here as concentric circles to emphasise that they are nested in one another. Each time frame contains the operations organized on shorter time scales and is contained by those with longer time scales (reproduced with permission from Kien and Altman 1995)

internal representation, when the choice collapses and a new selection can be made. The internal representations provide an essential reference or standard for determining whether the action should continue or is complete. They can be intrinsic to the structure of the system, such as membrane channels in neurons (Changeux) or synaptic connectivity, selected by evolution and development; and memories, continually sculpted by experience (Churchland). As CHOOSE-AND-COMPARE operates from moment to moment both within and between the time frames, it is the equivalent of the radius in Figure 2. This in turn represents the operations depicted by our ANN model (Fig. 1).

A common criticism of ANNs is that they tend to get stuck in one attractor, not a good model for the dynamic processes of decision-making! Klaus Nützel and colleagues in the Physics Department at the University of Regensburg, working in collaboration with Jenny Kien and me, have found modifications of ANN architecture that display dynamic behaviour very similar to that of motor nervous systems (Nützel et al. 1994). The three essentials are that connectivity in the network is low, asymmetrical and includes more than one value for "synaptic" delays. Even small networks with this architecture will relax into a robust but not rigid cyclical attractor, that is, visiting a stable sequence of states, but are also capable of spontaneously moving to a new sequence.

Both the time-frame and ANN models are intended for exploring the principles of functional architecture in the nervous system, rather than for simulation of experimental data. The time-frame model clarifies for experimentalists the temporal relationships between different organisational levels involved in the decision-making process. The networks provide simple systems for examining the computations that result in the selection of one sequence and not another, and for determining the conditions that allow a small change in input to precipitate a dramatic change in output. Together they may help us further along the road towards understanding how we decide what to do next.

Acknowledgments. Most of the research described in this chapter has been done in collaboration with Dr. Jenny Kien at the Institut für Zoologie, Universität Regensburg, Germany, and supported by the Deutsche Forschungsgemeinschaft through SFB4, project H-2. I also thank our colleagues in the Institut für Theoretische Physik, Regensburg, for their work in developing the dynamic ANN model.

References

Altman JS, Kien J (1987a) A model for decision making in the insect nervous system. In: Ali MA (ed) Nervous systems in invertebrates. Plenum, New York, 621–643

Altman JS, Kien J (1987b) Functional organization of the subesophageal ganglion in arthropods. In: Gupta AP (ed) Arthropod brain: its evolution, development, structure and functions. Wiley, New York, 265–301

Altman JS, Kien J (1989) New models for motor control. Neural Computation 1:173–183

Damasio AR (1994) Descartes' error. Emotion, reason, and the human brain. Putnam, New York. French trans.: l'erreur de Descartes. Odile Jacob, Paris

Kien J (1983) The initiation and maintenance of walking in the locust. An alternative to the command concept. Proc Roy Soc Lond B 219:137–174

Kien J, Altman JS (1992a) Decision making in the insect nervous system: a model for selection and maintenance of motor programmes. In: Kien J, McCrohan CR, Winlow W (eds) Motor programme selection: new approaches to the study of behavioural choice. Elsevier Science Ltd: Oxford, 147–169

Kien J, Altman JS (1992b) Preparation and execution of movement: parallels between insect and mammalian motor systems. Comp Biochem Physiol 103A:15–24

Kien J, Altman JS (1995) Modelling the generation of long-term neuronal activity underlying behaviour. Prog Neurobiol, 45:361–372

Kien J, McCrohan CR, Winlow W (eds) (1992) Motor programme selection: new approaches to the study of behavioural choice. Elsevier Science Ltd: Oxford

Kupfermann I, Weiss KR (1978) The command neuron concept. Behav Brain Sci 1:1–10

Nützel K, Kien J, Bauer K, Altman JS, Krey U (1994) Dynamics of diluted attractor neural networks with delays. Biol Cybern 70:553–561

Subject Index

Springer-Verlag
and the Environment

We at Springer-Verlag firmly believe that an international science publisher has a special obligation to the environment, and our corporate policies consistently reflect this conviction.

We also expect our business partners – paper mills, printers, packaging manufacturers, etc. – to commit themselves to using environmentally friendly materials and production processes.

The paper in this book is made from low- or no-chlorine pulp and is acid free, in conformance with international standards for paper permanency.

Printing: Saladruck, Berlin
Binding: Buchbinderei Lüderitz & Bauer, Berlin

DATE DUE